The Soul of a Patient

Lessons in Healing for Harvard Medical Students

Also by Susan E. Pories, MD, FACS

The Soul of a Doctor:
Harvard Medical Students Face Life and Death

Cancer: Biography of a Disease

Navigating Your Surgical Career: The AWS Guide to Success

The Soul of a Patient

Lessons in Healing for Harvard Medical Students

Edited by

Susan E. Pories, MD, FACS

Samyukta Mullangi, MD, MBA, Aakash Kaushik Shah, MD, and
Mounica Vallurupalli, MD

Gordian Knot Books

An Imprint of Richard Altschuler & Associates, Inc.

Laguna Woods, CA

Distributed by Ingram

The Soul of a Patient: Lessons in Healing for Harvard Medical Students. Copyright © 2018 by Susan E. Pories. For information or to arrange for special orders, contact the publisher, Gordian Knot Books, at (424) 279-9118, or send an email to Richard.Altschuler@gmail.com.

Library of Congress Control Number: 2018952895
CIP data for this book are available from the Library of Congress

ISBN-13: 978-1-884092-23-7

Gordian Knot Books is an imprint of
Richard Altschuler & Associates, Inc.

Cover Design: Sue Meyer

Printed in the United States of America

Distributed by Ingram

Dedication

For our families . . . There is no meaning in life without you.

Contents

Foreword by Jerome Groopman and Pamela Hartzband ix

Introduction by Susan E. Pories xi

Trust 1
Mother's Day by Ariel Wagner 3
Dimensions of a Secret Life by Samyukta Mullangi 9
Destiny by Manjinder Singh Kandola 18
Hoping for the Best, Preparing for the Worst by
    Mounica Vallurupalli 31

Revelations 39
Heartbeats by Galina Gheihman 41
Sacrifices by Ithan Peltan 80
Cheerful Bravado by Janine Knudsen 91
Taking Things as They Come by Carla Heyler 102

Acceptance 109
Beyond Alphabet Soup by Priyanka Saha 111
A Favorite Chair by Aakash Kaushik Shah 145
Invest in the Beginning by Kia Byrd 155
Like a Job by Aleks Olszewski 178
Vesuvius by Grace Lee 193
It Is What It Is by Ada Amobi 212

Understanding 223
The Diagnosis by Clare Malone 225
Infinity by Daniel Seible 233
Time for Questions by Davis "Mac" Stephen 258
Eight Percent by Morgan Prust 266
Reflections on a Journey by Eugene Vaios 285

Epilogue: Beginnings by Lisa Mayer, Nancy Oriol,
    Robert C. Stanton, and Katharine Treadway 305

About the Editors   313

Course Faculty   314

Student Authors   314

Acknowledgments   319

Foreword

JEROME GROOPMAN, MD and
PAMELA HARTZBAND, MD

Medical school is a time of learning. Traditionally in the first year, students are taught facts about anatomy, physiology and pharmacology. They sit for exams in these subjects, demonstrating that they have learned to identify specific nerves, muscles, bones and organs, and how these body parts function or fail to function. They learn how medications can augment or inhibit the workings of the body: the movement of blood through our vessels, electricity through our heart, water through our kidneys. In the first year, students are also introduced to patients at the bedside. There they learn the skills of physical examination, how to peer into the eyes and visualize the retina, palpate the breadth of the liver, assess the briskness of a limb's reflexes, and recognize what is normal and what is not.

As this collection shows, there is another kind of learning that occurs when students meet patients in that first year of medical school. It is a learning that goes beyond the physical assessment of the human body. It is an assessment of what we call mind and soul. The students probe the psychological and spiritual dimensions of a patient's life. Entry into these dimensions demands proficiency in how to listen, hear and understand. We witness in each of these narratives the journey of intelligent and motivated learners into a world that is new to them.

We see how the student's understanding draws not only on what a patient says but also on recognizing what is unsaid. They also learn how to read the subtleties of body language, to interpret a person's mien and posture as clues to his or her thoughts and emotions. The student becomes aware of how his or her own words and body language can communicate compassion and connection or apathy and disinterest. These doctors-in- training learn to explain to patients what may be the cause of their symptoms and what their prognosis may be, testing words that educate and comfort and words that fail to resonate.

Each story shows that the students learn that becoming an excellent clinician requires more than mere knowledge, more than the facts taught in the classroom about health and disease. They learn how to judiciously and compassionately apply that knowledge for the good of the individual patient—in diverse clinical conditions, including epilepsy, cystic fibrosis, ulcerative colitis, stroke, AIDS, breast cancer and heart failure. This, they realize, is the "art of medicine."

In each instance, the students turn inward, take their own emotional temperature and that of their patients, as they struggle to be a positive presence at the bedside. They summon feelings and ideas that come from their upbringing and their experiences, before entering the medical world. There is a core lesson that we take from the many stories recounted by a diverse class of young women and men in their first moments with their patients: To be both a doctor and a healer, they learn that they must deeply know themselves.

This, then, is a book of revelations, revealing how doctors learn to master their dual mission of care for the body and care for the soul. That learning begins in the first year of medical school, and extends throughout a physician's life.

Introduction

SUSAN E. PORIES, MD, FACS

There is nothing quite as important as training the next generation of physicians. In an increasingly complex and cruel world, finding a compassionate and skilled physician is truly a lifeline. Yes, of course we want our doctors to be up-to-date on all the latest medical knowledge and scientifically savvy; but, above all, we need physicians to be good listeners and caring practitioners.

Conceptualized by thoughtful educators at Harvard Medical School, the Mentored Clinical Casebook Project (MCCP) pairs a first-year medical student with a clinical mentor and a patient to follow closely for one year[1]. The student spends time with his or her patient, both in and out of clinical settings, with the goal of trying to understand the patient's life and relationship with his or her illness as completely as possible. The student keeps a written record of the interactions with the patient, and also does research to understand the scientific, socioeconomic, and cultural issues that influence the patient's experience.

The casebooks that are produced are quite impressive, some as long as ten thousand words, with extensive bibliographies and scientific tables. But what shines throughout is the singular relationships that these brand new students, not really doctors yet, forge with their patients. They go to appointments with them, have coffee, visit their homes, meet their families, and also meet the doctors caring for them. The students come away with a newfound appreciation for all sides of these complex situations. They have been assigned patients with chronic and sometimes terminal illness, and have the opportunity to witness the bravery and courage that facing these circumstances require.

We wanted to share these remarkable casebooks to shine a light on this innovative approach to medical education. Because the casebooks were so comprehensive, for this collection we decided to emphasize the personal struggles associated with illness and the connection and communication with the caregiver that is so important to patient-centered care. We took out details of the basic science and clinical care, because these change with new knowledge and techniques, while relationships and communication skills are timeless.

This collection of first-year medical students writing about their year-long experiences with patients is truly unique and inspiring. As a breast surgeon and medical educator, I learn something new every day from my patients and my students. Reading and editing these extraordinary casebooks with a team of talented student-editors has been a privilege and joy. I am thankful for the opportunity to share these with a larger audience.

[1.]Stanton, RC, Mayer, LD, Oriol, NE et al, Acad Med. 2007; 82:516.

TRUST

My ideal doctor would be my Virgil, leading me through my purgatory or inferno, pointing out the sights as we go. . . . Just as he orders blood tests and bone scans of my body, I'd like my doctor to scan *me*, to grope for my spirit as well as my prostate.

— Anatole Broyard, *Doctor, Talk to Me*

Mother's Day

ARIEL WAGNER

I begin the course filled with excitement and naiveté. Though I have no idea who my patient will be, I imagine us forming an instant bond. The relationship will imbue my otherwise dry basic science courses with purpose, I tell myself. I will take the time to listen and reflect, and I will become a better scribe for the patient experience. Even without knowing my patient, I know it will be perfect. It never occurs to me that it could be otherwise.

The first time I hear of Nidal, he is twelve years old and described to me as "vegetative." I jot this down on a Post-It note, along with his numerous other diagnoses. When I meet Nidal in the hospital, he lies prostrate in his hospital bed, eyes open but not seeing, his occasional movements without purpose or merely reflexive. He has been like this for a long time, perhaps always. I am overwhelmed, not so much by sadness or pity at the sight of a twelve-year-old in this state, but by a sense of bewilderment as to the purpose of all of this. What kind of life is this? Why work so hard to prolong a life that seems either indifferent to the world or in a state of potentially constant suffering? The answer to these questions depends on whether you see Nidal as someone who has an inner life, and knows the world in some way, or whether you see him as vegetative.

His mother, Sabirah, believes he can sense and feel. "I know his brain works," she tells me. "He has life in him, but people don't see it. She will tell you he likes a little juice on his tongue or the "Finding Nemo" movie playing on the flat screen above his bed. She speaks to him and believes that, on some level, he understands. And even the doctor admitted that Nidal's responses appeared to be "a higher level than reflexive," in particular his utterances, or vocalizations, and smiles. These interpersonal expressions suggest that Nidal does, at least at times, experience a level of consciousness. As I try to understand his experience, I realize I am really trying to understand his mother's attachment to him. At the end of the day, it doesn't matter whether Nidal fits this or that criteria. Truth is in the eye of the beholder, and all that really matters is what is true for Sabirah, because she is Nidal's mother and the one who takes care of him.

When Children's Hospital calls Dr. Bahir to let her know that Nidal's old medical records are available, I see this as an opportunity to get to know Nidal in a different way; to get a sense of him from the beginning and to see how he has come to be what he is now. What was he like when he was born? How had he changed? I already know part of the story—the c-section, the chromosomal abnormality, the two months in neonatal intensive care. But Sabirah and I haven't talked much about the intervening years, and since Dr. Bahir only became Nidal's doctor a year ago, she doesn't know much about his history either. So we start with the first file and pick up where Sabirah left off.

Following his birth, Nidal's doctors noted that his head was quite small. It was smaller than most newborns. This did not seem too concerning at the time, because, as a "preemie," his whole body was small. Indeed, he was smaller than most newborns by length and weight as well. But by five months, his head had barely grown, dropping him down to the bottom two percent of infants within his age group. His head was no longer proportional to his body size and his doctors began to refer to him as microcephalic, which is almost always associated with developmental delay. Despite his brain's lagging growth, Nidal did seem to be making some progress developmentally. At five months, his neurologist indicated that he was "alert and active" on examination. He could make cooing and other vowel sounds and was able to bring his hands to his mouth. By his mother's account, he could recognize his parents and brother, although

4

it is hard to know whether this was truly the case. At the same time, the neurologist noted that Nidal was only able to fix his gaze on an object occasionally and his eye movements often seemed random. He could grasp objects but not for any prolonged period of time. He did not laugh. She also noted that he was turning his head rapidly from side to side and moving his arms in a way that appeared "excessive" and "perhaps involuntary." How concerning these signs were considered is not mentioned in the note. Even so, the picture seems to be one of at least some progress.

Reading through these early notes, I start to picture Nidal a little better. I see him as a newborn, reaching and smiling; see him fix his eyes on his mother, just long enough to tell her that he knows her. I imagine his mother's hopes as Nidal's condition stabilizes and she takes him home. I can imagine how, in many moments, he seemed like any other newborn. The hopefulness is overshadowed, however, by the knowledge of what is to come. Eventually, the markers of progress seem to disappear. Nidal can't crawl or sit up. His vision worsens and he is determined to be blind. His seizures continue, despite medication. By the time I reach his files for early childhood, any neurological development that once existed appears to have halted.

Given all the difficulties Nidal faced as a child, I asked Sabirah if the doctors spoke to her about issuing a do not resuscitate order (DNR). Sabirah answers the question with emphasis. "We want everything," she tells me. Hoping to push her further, I ask her if she has always felt supported in this decision by Nidal's doctors and nurses. She pauses, clearly thinking it over. "I don't know if everyone supports it," she tells me, "but no one has ever been disrespectful." I am heartened and somewhat surprised, to hear this. After thinking about the question longer, memories of caretakers who clearly didn't see things her way return. Sabirah recalls an occasion when the nurses referred to Nidal as "comatose" after a hospitalization at Children's. "They didn't see him as a viable human being," she tells me. "They saw him as someone we were wasting good time and energy on that could have gone to other children." This statement resonates with me because it exactly articulates my own sentiments upon first meeting Nidal. I have whole journal entries devoted to this single thought. No matter how hard I tried to empathize and understand, I always came back to it. An almost incomprehensible amount of energy and resources, wasted on a child who couldn't benefit. It seemed so absurd and unfair.

One afternoon, while waiting for Sabirah, I find myself alone with Nidal in his hospital room. I attempt to reconcile my views on the energy and resources spent on him with those of his mother. As I sit there, I stare at him, trying to read his face, his body. I try to feel some connection to him, something to make me understand his mother's affection, to make me feel allied with him as my patient. That Nidal can't respond doesn't make him that different from many children I have cared for and to whom I have felt connected. Infants are unaware of themselves and unable to communicate except by crying, and yet I often felt a seemingly instant attachment to the infants I worked with in Mali. But I fail to develop a similar affinity for Nidal. I don't know why it doesn't come. So I just sit there. I watch him, I reflect, I wait for a connection, but it never comes.

When I look at Nidal, there are a lot of things I think I am supposed to feel: sadness, affection, sympathy, a desire for him to get better. But more than any of these things, I feel angry. I spent two years as a Peace Corps volunteer in Mali, watching children die. I used to keep a journal. Not the usual sort of thing, where you write about your day and your feelings. It was a journal of dead children. Determined not to forget them, I wrote their names, descriptions of who they were, how I knew them, why I loved them. Immersed in a culture in which it was unacceptable to show emotion, I poured my pain into my entries. As helpless as I felt in those moments, I told myself that some way, somehow, I would do something to change this. However, no matter how much I cared or how hard I worked, the entries continued to pile up: malaria, malnutrition, diarrhea. Simple diseases, cheap deaths. The contrast between the two realities is so stark, I have a hard time moving past it. Sometimes when I get home from visiting Nidal, all I want to do is cry.

The last time I meet with Sabirah before completing my casebook, she tells me she couldn't imagine her life without Nidal. She never had any doubt about keeping him when she was pregnant, and she certainly doesn't have any doubt now. In my meetings with Sabirah, occasionally I get a glimpse of what her life was like before his birth. She worked as a science teacher in Boston, and she tells great stories about her students and the stunts they pulled in class. She was happily married to Nidal's father, her second husband. Her pregnancy, in particular, sounds like a happy time. She smiles as she remembers how excited her son, Aafiya, was to be having a baby brother. Things changed once Nidal was born. His father couldn't accept his condition, believing it to be a curse. He was "devastated," she tells me. But what devastated her was that he could be disappointed by what God gave them. In her understanding of Islam, any child was a gift. "God gave me this child," she tells me. "This is my gift and I will do all I can to make him happy." But the Islam her husband knew had taught him that disability was a form of punishment from God. Their views were not easily reconciled and, not surprisingly, the toll on their marriage was significant.

Despite his wife's pleas for him to spend time with his son, Nidal's father spent most of his time in Philadelphia, where he had a business and where his first wife and six daughters lived. Although he telephoned Sabirah daily, sometimes crying on the phone, he only visited once a year. "He's deaf. He's blind. He can't feel anything," he once shouted at her. "He should die." Although Sabirah doesn't let her emotions show as she repeats these words, there is no escaping the pain they must have inflicted. The words cut like a knife. I play them over and over again in my mind, trying to imagine what it must have been like for her, loving her child as she does, to hear these words from her own husband.

Is there value in a life like Nidal's? Six months ago, I might have answered "no." Today, however, my response is different. There is value in Nidal's life. Not so much for himself—as I still have no evidence he is aware of himself or the world around him—but for others. For one, there are the countless doctors, nurses, residents, and medical students like myself who have learned at his bedside. "He's a physiology textbook," Dr. Bahir told me when she first introduced me. "There's nothing you can learn about the human body that Nidal can't teach you."

There are also the other disabled children and their families who benefit from Sabirah's advice and example. Indeed, she has become an advocate not only for her own son but for disabled children in general. Through her "Team Nidal" Facebook page, she shares information about his condition and her experience caring for him, not to mention an assortment of medical articles, prayers, and motivational thoughts she thinks may be of interest to other parents. That many who visit the site write to Sabirah for advice or to thank her for her words is just one indication of the impact she has had on the lives of others, an impact only possible through Nidal's inspiration.

Perhaps more important than any of this, however, is the role Nidal plays in his mother's life. While those on the outside may look at the two of them and be overwhelmed by the burden and the sacrifices required by his care, this is not what Sabirah sees. To her, Nidal is a source of happiness and love. He provides her life with meaning. And what is more valuable than that?

Dimensions of a Secret Life

SAMYUKTA MULLANGI

Most everyone would agree that, in this age of social media and online networking, it has become absurdly easy to know a great deal about a person before you even meet him. It only takes a couple of search terms in your Google taskbar, or some basic navigation through those ever dwindling degrees of separation in your Facebook friend circles, to find most anyone, and discover where they're from, their birthday, their alma mater, whether they like watching "30 Rock," and what they did last weekend. When it's this simple to mine this kind of information, I guess I shouldn't have been surprised to gain access to the secret life of my patient months before I even ever knew what he looked like.

And yet, I was.

I was taking an elective, during my first year as a Harvard medical student, called the Mentored Clinical Casebook Project. My mentor, Dr. Cutler, with the patient's permission, had given me his medical files to sift through in preparation for this meeting: progress notes, phone conversations, lab data. Just like that, I was made privy to the patient's information in a way that I had never had access to another human being before. I knew about his HIV and his last CD4 count, which measures the response to treatment for HIV (if effective, the count will increase). I knew something about his family, their health histories, and their private resentments. I knew about his first boyfriend. I even knew his IQ.

A few weeks later, I found myself seated at the neighborhood Starbucks, waiting for my patient, Larry, a shy man who did not possess a computer or a cell phone, and who lived in an assisted living community that didn't easily allow visitors.

We were meeting in a coffee shop patronized by everyone from the fresh-faced dental student studying tooth physiology over a cinnamon latte to the overworked endocrinology fellow downing a triple espresso-shot by the counter. I was two weeks into my clinical epidemiology and health policy courses, both of which suddenly seemed so dry and impersonal to me in comparison.

Yet, as I sat there alone, waiting, I already felt invested in my patient. Though Harvard was doing an admirable job at exposing first-year students to the wards, and to interviewing patients on a weekly basis, we never really got to engage with our patients beyond the questions on our checklist. We acquainted ourselves with sets of questions that targeted body parts, symptoms, and social issues with tenacity. But, we were role-playing at being something we were not. Medical school had mobilized a sense of self-estrangement in us. In the wake of admissions interviews, we were convinced, as was everyone around us, that we knew exactly why we wanted to practice medicine; we thus found ourselves in a situation where we realized we knew nothing at all, actually, but still had to keep the pretense up. We were expected to enter a hospital room in our short white coats, shake hands confidently, and interview a patient with the objective of convincing everyone watching that, even in the absence of context, we could get the script down.

Though I appreciated the practicality driving the clinical interview, I found myself wondering how something as complex and vast as the world of medicine could be distilled into a set of simple questions. Did the pain radiate? Was the cough wet or dry? I knew to gently ask whether the patient felt safe at home, but could only pass him or her off to an imaginary social worker if the reply was not in the affirmative. The questions seemed too limited and too simple.

My preceptor emphasized that, at our level of training, the point of these interactions wasn't to learn the diagnosis, per se, but to learn how to build a relationship with a patient. The diagnosis and the relationship had been presented to us, first-year students, as mutually exclusive concepts: when in pursuit of one, we inevitably gave less importance to the other. Larry would be the first patient with whom I was going to be given the opportunity to marry the two.

We were sipping hot chocolate. The November air outside was pleasantly mild, surprising for the trend of miserably cold days that we had been experiencing lately. I would soon learn that he was particularly sensitive to the weather. He would often cancel our meetings when the temperature dipped below 50 degrees.

Larry was sitting across from me, and he stared warily at the number of sheets in front of me: one that held a list of questions, one where I scribbled down his current medical issues in shorthand, and a few blank papers for taking notes. I pointedly pushed them slightly away, and asked him to tell me about his life.

"Tell me about your childhood," I said.

It was then that his face darkened a bit. "Oh, I was a klutz at sports," he said. "I was bullied in high school." A pause. "Children can very cruel, you know."

I nodded. "Yes"

Over the course of the year, as I got to know him better, I continued to be impressed by his three-dimensionality, his "divided self" (as our professor Arthur Kleinman would call it), his insistence on defying my preconceptions about his life. He really liked his doctor and felt as though having these periodic conversations with me was the least he could do to pay the doctor back for his care. "But why are you doing this project?" he wanted to know.

If the patient's medical life and social life comprised the first component of our 3-D relationship, the second was my own history. This narrative would be incomplete without describing why I chose to take this class, and why I wanted to follow a patient with HIV. My family lived in India for the better part of my first sixteen years, with one brief interlude in the United States, as my father pursued a fellowship at the Mayo Clinic in the early nineties. I grew up for most of my life in a small town in the state of Andhra Pradesh in south India. My mother was an obstetrician and gynecologist for a Swiss missionary hospital. To add to her somewhat meager pay, the hospital gave us the luxury of living in a large bungalow at the edge of its campus, where a row of six such houses constituted the doctor's quarters. Alongside my family, there was a pediatrician, a general surgeon, and an infectious disease specialist in our neighborhood, residing with their families.

To say that I grew up surrounded by medicine is an understatement. It was the stuff of the usual for my sister and I to be picked up by a rickshaw *wallah* at 7:30 in the morning in front of our house, and to be cycled past the morning cohort of Catholic nuns and nurses, in white uniform, tending to the multitudes of people thronging the hospital's longitudinally laid out campus, to be seen by the doctor as soon as possible. On our other side rushed a wide, moss-flavored tributary of the Krishna River, separated from the hospital's campus by a cross-ratcheted metal fence. We always cycled past the small chapel where the nuns held morning and evening services, a homely building with a tapered roof that looked like it was plucked straight out of a German children's book. We would pass these peculiar sights every morning and then after school; these were our favorite places for play during the weekends. This was the storybook setup of my childhood. When our rickshaw swept through the front gates of the hospital and into the real world, it could feel absolutely jarring. The difference in the fragrant, clean, green, and seductively strange world of the hospital campus, and that of the brown, grimy, crowded and loud world of the rest of the town could not be greater.

Growing up in small town India in the nineties was like growing to adulthood in a secluded, closed-up, tied-away part of the world that could be as confining and hush-hush as one needed it to be. It seems bizarre to think back to those days now, as I type into my MacBook Pro, while listening to Chopin on Pandora, and flitting between the *New York Times*, the *New Yorker*, and the *New England Journal of Medicine* web pages with ease, instantly accessing a cornucopia of information about the world in a matter of seconds; to remember a time when we didn't have a computer or cable television, where the daily newspaper that we had delivered was written in Telugu (a language I could speak fluently but not read as well), and to think that I spent most of my formative years thus completely in the dark about the rest of the world; to recall that I finally had to learn to type by enrolling in a secretarial school, where I practiced the QWERTY keyboard by punching letters into ancient typewriters too heavy and deep for my eleven-year-old fingers; to think that I had never had a health class in all my years of schooling in India, to never have known what sex really entailed until I was well into my mid-teens, to have been informed about menarche one month before I actually experienced it, that my classmates, in step with the political rhetoric of the day, actually believed that homosexuality was a figment of the Western culture; and for HIV to mean very little to us.

I still remember those early conversations between my parents that I overheard, when they were discussing details about operating on HIV positive patients, and not understanding the complexity of the issue. I remember the advertisements featuring Balbir Pasha, the eponymous Indian character, whose story was narrated in a variety of television and print ads via song and dance. He was the fictional young man who didn't protect himself from HIV and was now infected. If Balbir Pasha could get infected, any of us could. But problems still abounded. There were still reports of infected children being forcibly expelled from schools, of harassment towards those whose status was disclosed at the workplace, and of raped girls now being doubly discriminated against—one for the crime of being raped and one for the possibility of being infected. The Shiv Sena, a Hindu nationalist party with deeply Marxist and religious sentiments, began to issue war cries against anything that smelled remotely Western—from McDonalds to public displays of affection, from homosexuality to HIV.

I applied to the Mentored Clinical Casebook Project with a firm vision of what I wanted from the endeavor. I wanted to be matched with someone who was HIV positive. I wanted to put a face to the disease that I had heard encountered on two continents with two very different but changing social and moral frameworks.

After one series of cancelled meetings, I began to wonder whether Larry was experiencing a resurgence of depression. The disease had been alluded to in previous notes by his therapist. I asked Dr. Cutler if there was a medical connection between HIV and psychiatric issues. I had heard that AIDS dementia was one of the effects of the virus on the body. "Perhaps that's not the way to understand them," he said. "In my experience, it is often the underlying psychiatric disorders, like anxiety, depression, PTSD and bipolar disorder that cause you to engage in behaviors that put you at risk for HIV." For instance, if someone was depressed, he or she may find solace in sex and drugs. These behaviors would then put that person at risk for contracting HIV.

Dr. Cutler saw my patient's issues as very different from those of someone experiencing the slow, cognitive decline from HIV. He saw more of a role for the absence of social networks and supportive relationships, a theme that he says is very prevalent in the gay community, and especially to the subset of those who are also beset with HIV. "In the past, coming out meant leaving many of his friends behind. HIV just amplifies these social problems," he noted. "For those who become addicts, it's more complicated. It's something they're not proud of and don't want people to know about. It can be depressing."

I sat back as Dr. Cutler treated me to the best kind of history of medicine: his personal memories of the emergence of HIV in San Francisco.

In 1996, there was a huge change in the AIDS story, in its very culture. Prior to this, there were only a couple of therapies on the market that would block viral multiplication during an opportunistic infection crisis. But there wasn't much of a survival benefit; rather, the treatments were analogous to chemotherapy in the context of metastatic disease. No cure, just buying time.

Then in 1996, protease inhibitors were introduced and the treatment of AIDS evolved from using single drugs to a more potent combination of several medications. "Before '96, there was an insurance industry that flourished in neighborhoods like Castro, where there were a lot of gay men. These companies would buy your life insurance policy from you and make you a deal," Dr. Cutler explained, his tone still marveling at the memory. "They'd get your million when you passed, and give you something like $700K right then, so that way you would get cash before you die, and they would turn a profit.

That business just does not exist anymore for people with HIV. Then, there were all these counter-stories about people who built up crazy credit card bills because they were, like, screw it, I'm going to die, but then they survived on and had to figure it out."

Dr. Cutler paused and smiled.

"Everybody just started living."

It took a couple of years for people to be sure that change was actually real. Was this just a delay in death or was it really long term survival? It soon became clear that it was the latter. According to Dr. Cutler, it is the same idea that applies to care now. In 1996, the crisis was over in SF in a very real way.

"If you imagined a community where a third of people have diabetes, it would be a big problem, right? After '96, it was still not trivial, still a big deal, but all these folks went out and began doing different things—writing, filmmaking, consulting.

"In the 1990s, care had already gotten a lot better. We had antibiotics to prevent pneumonia, for example. But still, all these people have HIV, and they're all going to die. An older colleague told me that he stopped counting the people who died at two hundred. I always wondered, why two hundred?"

I stop taking notes for a moment while I look at Dr. Cutler, and he continues to think aloud. Then he collects himself. "If you look through history, these kinds of big events influence people for the rest of their lives even though these events are long gone." Doctors get into treating tuberculosis or cancer because someone in the family had one of these diseases, he notes. "It was more like, here was this world where this disease had just *transformed* people."

I remember telling Dr. Cutler that I wanted to follow a young female with HIV. Instead, I got a male senior citizen, who disdains modern conveniences like cell phones and email, frequently cancelled coffee dates with me, blaming his seasonal affective disorder, and once asked me to make a home visit, despite having just told me that he lived in a dangerous neighborhood, right across the street from "a house of ill-repute."

Yes, Larry is quite the character. Though I would like to think that my friendship with him was worthwhile to him and his time, it has definitely meant a lot to me. It isn't just that I have been able to observe how HIV care has changed from acute crisis type of care to what Dr. Cutler analogizes to diabetes care. It isn't that I have learned how to competently do the medical interview, patiently listen, and quietly support.

It's all that and more. Larry completely upended my notions of the doctor-patient relationship, and made me so acutely aware of the fact that an individual's interiority is, as Arthur

Kleinman beautifully put it, split and discordant. He taught me that there is no one more real, more interesting, or more relevant than the person sitting across from you, be it at Starbucks or at the clinic. He taught me to be less cynical, to invest in people, and to reflect more, and deeply.

For I am now struck, as Gabriel Garcia Marquez's captain, by the "suspicion that it is life, more than death, that has no limits." And I am much better for it.

Destiny

MANJINDER SINGH KANDOLA

There was considerable energy in the room that morning, significantly more than there had been over the last few days. After the first few weeks of medical school, the wide grins and excited chatter had begun to die down, as the chilly breeze in Boston began to signal the upcoming winter, and the never-ending biochemistry lectures pointed to a long year ahead.

But this morning was different. We were scheduled to meet an actual patient. We were told that the patient had multiple myeloma (a blood cancer formed by malignant plasma cells), and that we would have the opportunity to see the drugs we had been learning about in class in an applied clinical setting. The peptide structures and arrows were to become real, the hypothetical case scenarios and simulations suddenly brought to life. The transformation of the lecture hall was remarkable. The ties had returned, seats were once again filled, and classmates that I hadn't seen since the first day of school were sitting in the very front, eager not to miss a single word of the discussion. We were eventually introduced to Dr. Lennon, an esteemed clinician and researcher at the Cancer Center just down the street. His dynamic presence, his glowing face, and his genuine smile immediately eclipsed the uncommonly vibrant energy in the room. He began to teach us about multiple myeloma, responsible for eleven thousand deaths a year. We learned that cancerous cells are actually characterized by abnormal and abundant growth. In this case, plasma cells, necessary for the production of antibodies and a healthy immune system, begin to reproduce uncontrollably and put out abnormal proteins, resulting in bone lesions, anemia, fatigue and weakness, and potentially even serious kidney damage.

Dr. Lennon was a gifted storyteller, and he told us the clinical course of thalidomide, a drug patented in the mid-twentieth century and marketed for the treatment of respiratory infections. Researchers soon realized that the drug had anti-nausea properties that helped treat conditions of morning sickness, and it became incredibly popular and widespread. But just as suddenly, pregnant women taking the drug began giving birth to children with severe growth deformities, and usage plummeted. An Israeli physician later discovered its useful effects against a skin complication of leprosy, and interestingly, it was later discovered to have significant effects on the immune system, allowing it to be a potent treatment against multiple myeloma. Dr. Lennon was only getting started. He shifted gears to talk about a new medication marketed under the trade name Velcade, the newest and most effective therapy at the time for newly diagnosed patients with multiple myeloma. This medication blocks the growth of the tumor cells. And just like that, a disease that once carried such a tragic prognosis and was linked to just a few years of survival was witnessing a significant transformation in treatment. Patients, who once could only be treated with infusions of healthy blood cells (stem cell transplants) along with toxic high-dose drugs that suppressed the immune system, suddenly had tangible treatment options. Living with the disease for at least a decade was becoming far less unusual.

With beaming optimism, Dr. Lennon introduced us to our clinical case for the morning. Tom was a delicate and frail man, but if there was anyone who looked even more hopeful than Dr. Lennon, it was he. He wasn't alone. His wife came and sat right next to him, symbolic of the long and difficult journey they had taken together in battling Tom's myeloma. Tom was one of the few patients who had managed to survive with the disease for so long, especially given the relatively primitive treatment options that were available at the time of his diagnosis. Unfortunately, the rapid rate of tumor growth allows for resistance to develop against many of the drugs that we use.

Even though most tumor cells can be eradicated with toxic therapy, even a small percentage of resistant cells can repopulate the entire cancer. And, indeed, he had gone through several rounds of remission and relapse. Each time, his health had declined due to side effects of these therapies, and Dr. Lennon explained that treatment with thalidomide had caused peripheral neuropathy, or damaged nerve signaling to Tom's limbs. Unfortunately, he was likely to have another relapse in the near future.

As I looked at Tom, I couldn't help but wonder how he could remain so brave and hopeful, after dealing with so many ailments through repeated rounds of treatment and relapse. And it wasn't just physically taxing. The emotional burden seemed insurmountable, as I sat there with tears in my eyes just from listening to the story. How could he have so much courage, knowing the cancer would relapse, knowing he would just have to do it all over again?

The support that he had was clearly an incredibly important factor. As he clenched his wife's hand, he remarked, "She is everything to me." She was the reason that he continued to fight, and the reason that he could. And the other factor was the relationship he had with his physician. When someone asked Tom how he dealt with the mental challenge of taking so many different drugs, especially when many of them were still experimental and were only speculated to be useful treatments, he confidently said, "I'll take anything and everything that Dr. Lennon gives me. He knows what's best." The physician-patient bond that we had so often heard about from our faculty was right in front of our eyes.

I suddenly knew why Tom seemed so special. My dad was diagnosed with hepatitis C roughly 20 years ago, at around 40 years of age. He had two young kids, was the only working member of an immigrant family, and struggled to make ends meet for all of us. He had yet to experience any symptoms of the disease. His doctor, who was also Indian, explained that hepatitis C often lies dormant in the liver for long stretches of time, and that he had likely gotten it back in India, where reusing needles in clinics was all too common while he was growing up. His doctor then referred him to a specialist, whom my dad asked what it would take to cure the disease. The doctor spoke English, creating a slight language barrier, and explained that the drugs would have to be taken over at least a year, and that side effects included anything from depression to even suicide. My dad adamantly felt that taking medication that could lead to suicide, and to leave behind his entire family would be an utterly foolish thing to do, especially considering the costs of the treatment and the fact that he wasn't experiencing any symptoms at all from the disease. Nobody spoke of his hepatitis again.

A few years later, my dad, by chance, went back to his Indian physician, who asked him how things had gone with the hepatitis therapy. When my dad candidly told him what happened, his doctor was essentially stupefied. He very clearly explained to my dad that the side-effects were rare, and for someone who had such a strong support network from his family, he would definitely be able to get through his treatment. My brother and I didn't really understand his disease at the time, but he told us everything would be all right, and after talking it over with my mom, decided to go through with the treatment.

Sure enough, his life was absolutely awful for the next year. I saw him struggle to tie his turban in the morning, but he would say that he had no choice but to go to work. He was fatigued all the time and started to become irritable, which I had never seen before from the man who once responded with patience and a smile, no matter the situation. The drugs damaged his liver and his thyroid gland, and he even had to be hospitalized a few times. But he never gave up, and it was his relationship with his family and his physician that gave him the courage to continue on. It was the very support that I was seeing now with Tom.

Class had ended, but I was hooked. I continued to think about Tom and Dr. Lennon, and how a physician could form such a strong bond with his patients. I immediately wrote to Dr. Lennon, asking him if I could come and shadow him sometime and experience first-hand what these interactions must be like. And he happily agreed.

The very first time I met Dr. Lennon in clinic, he told a story from the time he visited a close friend in India. The two of them were on the way back from dinner with a Sikh family when their rickshaw driver accidentally hit a pedestrian. As the pedestrian lay injured and the two of them tried to gather their thoughts and help the injured man, the driver fled the scene. Suddenly a mob began to assemble, suspecting that the outsiders had harmed their fellow villager. Dr. Lennon and his friend tried to explain what had really happened, but it was to no avail. The villagers began to become increasingly hostile, knives were drawn, and Dr. Lennon remarked, "I didn't think we would make it out of there that day." After a brief pause, his glowing smile quickly returned, and he reassured me that his Sikh friend had gotten word of what was happening and immediately came to their rescue. The man was quite respected among the other villagers, and their trust in his word quickly quelled the situation.

Trust. What is trust, really? The word gets thrown around all the time, especially early in our training as aspiring physicians. "You must forge a bond of trust with your patients." "Trust is a two-way street." I had heard countless clichés revolving around this pervasive and yet elusive concept. But interestingly enough, my most formative experiences regarding trust actually came from meeting patients in whose journeys it had been explicitly lacking. But I was at the Cancer

Center's multiple myeloma clinic, one of the world's best providers of high-quality care for this disease. It was the intersection of esteemed faculty, the newest drugs, and highly motivated patients. Trust must come easily for them, I thought.

My initial thoughts weren't entirely unfounded. "I'm excited to introduce you to this patient, Manjinder. He comes all the way from India," Dr. Lennon remarked one afternoon. Indeed, I was now faced with a man who had traveled all the way from Hyderabad, India, with his wife, to receive a stem cell transplant for his condition, under the direction of one of the world's prominent myeloma experts. My cultural heritage helped me connect with this family, and I could see their faces light up as they saw me walk into the room, reassured that I might be someone with whom they could connect. After we talked about the difficulty in transitioning to a completely new culture and environment, I asked him why he didn't elect to simply receive the transplant in India, where he was being otherwise well treated for his condition. Dr. Lennon pointed out that the post-transplant care in India might be less ideal for this gentleman given the risks involved, and that the experience of his care team here would go a long way in making sure he received the best care possible, a view which the patient and his family clearly agreed. He innocently said "*Salaam*" and "*Shukria*" as he walked out.

For the first time, I genuinely felt like I was part of the care team. I obviously defined my role to the patients that I talked to, but they still relayed their sincere concerns and questions with me. They passionately shared their experiences with their cancer, and I felt honored to partake in the journey with them. I was eternally grateful to them for extending such a tremendous privilege, and yet it was they who would thank me each and every time. "You're going to be an amazing doctor one day," many would say. It definitely circles back to trust. They trusted Dr. Lennon, and they knew he trusted me, and I suddenly shared in this incredible bond. It wasn't easy. With trust comes attachment, and I found myself caring very deeply about these patients that I had just met. I soon realized that part of the reason I felt so strongly attached was because of vulnerability. As patients relayed their fear and anxiety, they made themselves incredibly vulnerable, and evoked in me a passion to care for and about them. Trust. It is a physician's most powerful tool, but perhaps also just as dangerous. Patients can be incredibly vulnerable, and a physician's word or even sigh of relief can go a long way in influencing their thoughts and feelings. At the same time, we must be mindful that patients' faith in their physicians gives our thoughts and reflections incredible weight.

By the time I met Ron, I had interviewed many patients and was certainly starting to develop some sort of diagnostic intuition. We had just learned about diagnostic momentum, and the idea that it is quite common for physicians to take previous analysis and diagnosis at face value, with an unconscious bias that reinterprets any future symptoms in the context of this previous label. We were taught to consider every possibility, and to keep in mind previous diagnoses, but certainly not to be limited by them. I wondered to what extent our visual senses might also play a part in this. There is no question that just seeing a patient leads us to characterize his or her health in some way. However, these signs have generally been at least somewhat predictive, and they therefore aren't necessarily an error, but rather something to be mindful of. If that was indeed the case, things certainly didn't bode too well for Ron. He looked pale and fatigued, as he sat hunched over on the chair. He extended his hand to meet me and greeted me with an incredibly warm smile, but his eyes looked dejected. His arms were crossed, as if he needed energy to just hold them up. But he spoke slowly and confidently, with strength and courage.

Speaking to Ron confirmed my intuitions. He spoke of being diagnosed with degenerative disc disease several years ago, which required several surgeries and eventually caused him to be dismissed from his job. He had been the vice president of a large company, and aside from the ensuing financial burden, he had lost a job that he was passionate about, a job he had put his heart and soul into. Ron was a fighter, and he didn't give up. He began working odd jobs, and he had currently just started as a part-time retailer at a furniture store. In his spare time, he drove with Uber, trying to make ends meet.

But Ron was tired all the time. He barely had enough energy to wake up in the morning and put his clothes on. And, in this most vulnerable time, he and his wife were going through a divorce, which was emotionally exhausting for him, not to mention all of the court proceedings and lawyers who needed to be involved. "It's on good terms," he insisted. "We're still friends." It was in the midst of his financial distress and divorce, which led him to leave his home and daughters, and his emotional and physical fatigue, that he awaited a diagnosis of multiple myeloma. Dr. Lennon had been monitoring his protein levels for the past few years, which had recently started to trend upwards.

Ron was already dealing with mild fatigue, caused by anemia, but his clinical symptoms were not yet severe enough to warrant a full diagnosis. It certainly felt conflicting that we needed Ron to get a bit worse before he could get better. Dr. Lennon had been ever-monitoring his rising protein levels, anticipating his crossing the threshold that would allow us to treat his likely cancer. It was a ticking clock, and all we could do was wait. I would never have thought that I might want a patient's cancer to progress. And yet, as the three of us sat in the room, there was a hint of disappointment, as we realized that Ron's blood reports indicated that his myeloma diagnosis remained as "smoldering," an early step in the cancer before it became more malignant and harmful. It was good news, but at the same time, we could not justify the need to use medications that were still under study, and the most we could do was, therefore, to keep him under close supervision.

After Ron's physician left the room, speaking to him alone told a completely different story. He did, indeed, feel sick, but the ramifications of the treatment we hoped to implement suddenly became all too clear. "I feel like I'm drowning. I'm not ready to start any kind of treatment right now," he said. "I need to keep working my two jobs to provide for my family," he continued. And "I don't want anything to get in the way of my daughter's graduation." It was autumn and his daughter was graduating in the upcoming spring.

I suddenly began to wonder why we had hoped to push treatment in the first place. We were only trying to help, but hearing his perspective made us appear perhaps overly aggressive and controlling. As Ron kept talking, however, I realized that the myeloma did not come without serious and potentially life-threatening consequence. He had previously suffered serious bone damage, and degeneration of his spine caused significant back pain, although this was not from his myeloma and might, therefore, be difficult to distinguish from profession of disease. Inability to walk had caused him to lose his job of twelve years as vice president of a large company. Sometimes he could barely get out of bed and move in the mornings, due to muscle weakness. And yet things only seemed to be getting worse, despite the fact that his myeloma appeared quite stable. If there was one thing that Ron still had going for himself, it was that he was in the right place. The Cancer Center was leading a novel trial for the treatment of multiple myeloma.

Perhaps the most striking thing that Ron said was his remark that he felt like he was "drowning." I recently had a chance to see the Japanese Exhibit at the MFA, which featured Katsushika Hokusai's "The Great Wave off Kanagawa," which truly shed light on what Ron had said. It was interesting to see how apparent and majestic Mount Fuji was in every single work across the gallery, perhaps representing its ever-looming presence in the Japanese landscape. And yet, in the midst of the tumultuous scenery in this painting, it seems entirely unimportant. For the viewer is drowning.

Indeed, the novel treatment was analogous to Mount Fuji for us. It could save his life! How could he possibly be thinking about anything else? Perhaps one can't in serene waters. But Ron had lost his job, and left his home. He felt incredibly dispirited that it was tough to have his daughters over in his small apartment. "I have to find a place to live," he insisted. "And I just started my new job. How could I possibly tell them that I need time off?" he asked. The new job was part-time, and it certainly wasn't enough to cover his needs, but it was still something, and the treatment would get in the way. Dr. Lennon had reassured him that we were flexible with the schedule, that many of the other enrolled patients had jobs as well. Then there was his daughter's graduation, coming up in June. "I can't let anything get in the way of that!" he exclaimed. Myeloma was the last thing on Ron's mind. Ron helped me understand the substantial extent to which the journey against a disease like myeloma is mental, emotional, social, and rooted in one's support networks.

The sunshine peered in through the windows and brightened the room that Tuesday afternoon. The academic year was coming to an end, and I was looking forward to seeing Ron again. He was still concerned about his work situation, and said that driving for Uber barely drew a positive margin when considering the depreciation on his car—the same car in which he and his wife had just driven back from their final divorce proceeding. "It was a quiet ride back," he reflected. He was happy, though, that his daughter had gotten into nursing school and was graduating, and this seemed to bring them together. "I don't know how I'm going to pay for her tuition," he said.

The last time I saw Ron, he relayed his concerns with starting treatment. And yet he seemed hesitant to fully share his thoughts with Dr. Lennon. "We'll start you as soon as you're ready," Dr. Lennon said, as warmly as ever, as Ron nodded. But Dr. Lennon was referring to his clinical findings, which did not yet fit the inclusion criteria for the study. Ron lightly mentioned his concerns, and Dr. Lennon was optimistic, promising that we would find a way to work with them in a way to help him. And we left the conversation at that.

When he was finally eligible to be enrolled, he wasn't ready just yet. His daughter's graduation was coming up in June, and there was no chance that he would even consider therapy until after then. I wondered if it simply served to help him justify pushing it off further. Dr. Lennon completely understood, and reflected that they were willing to wait as long as it took, but cautioned that he should start as soon as possible. The exchange seemed reasonable enough, but was certainly off-putting. "What are the risks of holding off on treatment?" I asked Dr. Lennon later. "Well there's risk of end-organ failure and more advanced disease," he said. "So we will need to monitor him very carefully."

I felt incredibly uneasy. We had been learning all year about patient autonomy, and treating to meet the needs of the patient, but I couldn't help but feel disappointed. It was a frustration with the world that such a sincere and humble man didn't have access to potentially life-saving treatment. It was available but the social and financial issues surrounding Ron's life had made it too difficult for him to elect to have treatment at that point in time.

Seeing "The Wave" provided a powerful image to really understand my feelings regarding Ron's situation. It wasn't enough to just point at Mount Fuji and expect him to forget about everything else. I remember listening to a classmate say that patients aren't arrows that we can simply shoot towards the correct target; rather, they are birds with wings, and if we throw them, they will simply fly away. We have to truly motivate them and encourage them to fly towards the destination, if we expect to have any success. Such was the case with Ron, who was, in fact, drowning.

I loosened my tie as I walked out of the Cancer Center's glass walls, my mind buzzing with so many thoughts. It is interesting that we often think of access to health care as simply being a question of health insurance and having the means to acquire the treatment itself. Less discussed and understood are the structural barriers to other dimensions of care that remain as relevant as ever. We have to advocate for our patients, and that obligation extends far beyond the clinic walls. Each situation tremendously colors the patient interview, even though the fundamental set of questions remains the same. And it is precisely this diversity that makes this field so magical and wonderful. Each time I ask "What brings you here today?" I am genuinely curious and excited for the journey that I have the privilege to embark on next.

Originating in India five hundred years ago, the Sikh religion considers the pursuit of social and political justice the primary goal of each and every human being. It takes the concept of Western autonomy much further, declaring that we are all divine and individually sovereign. In one fell swoop, centuries of a deeply entrenched caste system and rooted patriarchal hegemony were conceptually lifted. We have a responsibility to protect the justice of others and in doing so, achieving freedom for ourselves.

It was the faith of the oppressed, and countless Sikhs have happily become martyrs since in the struggle for justice. One of the most powerful shabads, or sacred hymns in the Sikh tradition, reads along the lines of "Let me die such a death, that I shall never have to die again." Many interpret the shabad in the context of reincarnation, the cycle of rebirth among many Eastern schools of thought. The cycle itself is in many faiths considered a cycle of suffering, and achieving freedom from the cycle is thus the ultimate goal. The fifth guru of the Sikh tradition, Guru Arjun Dev Ji, who spent his life preaching these Sikh ideals, which were so revolutionary at the time, was called by the Muslim Emperor to the palace court, and ordered to be executed for his views that called for religious freedom. In an effort to erode his integrity, the court offered him a chance to live if he were to convert to the Muslim faith. He peacefully objected, agreeing to a particularly torturous death, which involved sitting in a boiling pot while having burning sand poured over his ulcerating body. A renowned Muslim priest, horrified at the actions of the court, ran to the guru and pleaded that he remain alive, to whom the guru responded that God's doings were sweet to him. He at last breath uttered the above-mentioned hymn as he passed away.

My recent experiences have completely transformed my interpretation of this hymn—for it is not about dying but, rather, about living. Reincarnation, which warns of living through animal life, is perhaps an elegant metaphor for the humanity that we lose when we don't struggle for justice. If we enslave ourselves, we have failed to recognize our own humanity, and risk wasting this divine human life. For Tom, achieving mental and emotional victory against his cancer gave him life. For Ron, the best treatment in the world had yet to do so, but we were reassured by the fact that it would be there when he was ready.

Let us not forget the many patients that pass away on their deathbeds happy, finally feeling free. It is in fighting for social justice and in our own courage and passion that we achieve true life and happiness, embracing our humanity. In rising above the fear of death, we achieve immortality.

Hoping for the Best, Preparing for the Worst

MOUNICA VALLURUPALLI

Leslie was being admitted to the hospital once again. This hospitalization was the most recent episode in her sixteen-year battle, punctuated by uncertainty and bolstered by hope, of living with cystic fibrosis, a progressive disease that causes persistent lung infections and breathing problems as well as difficulty absorbing food. She looked much younger than sixteen, drowning in a large gray sweatshirt. Her thin frame convulsed and startled me each time she shook with a fit of coughing.

Leslie's struggles with cystic fibrosis and the complications associated with its treatments are unique. But her illness has an ancient pedigree, one that geneticists have traced back over fifty thousand years to Stone Age Europe. This disease has persisted because the abnormal gene that causes it has been passed down from generation to generation. In the normal situation, the body produces a protein that helps to maintain a balance of salt and water in the pancreas and lungs. When the protein is defective it causes patients with cystic fibrosis to have excess salt in their sweat. Folklore in the Middle Ages foretold death for the child who tasted salty when kissed.

"She was such a small, fussy baby," explained her mother, a gregarious woman with large, thick-rimmed glasses and a hearty laugh. Much to Leslie's embarrassment, her mother explained how Leslie was diagnosed—recounting that she had the "worst smelling poop as a baby." As she was weaned from breastfeeding, she began to lose weight and continued to do so for several months. A battery of tests revealed her diagnosis of cystic fibrosis and her life was forever altered.

Over the next few hours, as Leslie waited for test results to come back, she distracted herself by making bead bracelets that she sold to raise money for the Cystic Fibrosis Foundation.

Just as I was about to leave, her nurse entered and told Leslie that her cough was due to a viral infection with "RSV" (respiratory syncytial virus). Her mom asked, with a tone that barely hid her concern, "Isn't this what Leslie had the last time she rejected." When I asked her mom about RSV, Leslie interjected, "It's Respiratory 'Sucky' Virus." In fact, it was Leslie's initial experience with "Respiratory Sucky Virus" that led to the rejection of her first lung transplant.

The life of a child with severe cystic fibrosis is dotted with frequent medical appointments, daily doses of a kaleidoscope of pills, careful nutrition monitoring, regular physical therapy, and the often unavoidable hospitalizations for lung infections. Sometimes, all of these interventions may not be enough, and once exhausted the only option that remains for patients with worsening lung function is a lung transplant—an option that Leslie had to consider earlier than most cystic fibrosis patients. By the time she was in fifth grade, Leslie had to take a tank of oxygen with her wherever she went. With her indefatigable *joie de vivre*, she attempted to learn to ride a bike with an oxygen tank strapped on. Yet, as her disease progressed and her lung function declined, she could no longer even climb the stairs in her home or take a shower without being breathless. Transplantation was her only solution.

It was not a decision she or her family came to easily. Prior to her first transplant, Leslie was given a packet to explain what to expect. Sixty-seven pages long, double spaced and written in an eerily friendly Comic Sans typeface, it explains in simple terms topics like "how do lungs work," "the transplant evaluation process," "complications after surgery," and "talking to the donor family."Leslie took the initiative in asking questions and seeking information about the process.

Once cleared for a lung transplant, each individual receives a score that ranks patients based on the severity of their illness. Children under the age of twelve, however, are ranked according to the time they have been waiting for a transplant. The pamphlet states, "Most often it is the waiting that is the most difficult and stressful for our patients." The wait, in Leslie's case, was agonizingly long, almost four years for her first transplant.

Leslie hoped that her transplant would allow her to be a normal kid who could breathe, swim, and ride a bike. But, even though she knew that a lung transplant was exchanging one diagnosis for another, it was a shock for her to realize all that she had to do to prevent rejection. It meant wearing a mask wherever she went, taking up to twenty pills a day in addition to managing her diabetes, pancreatic insufficiency, and checking her lung function as well as vital signs at least two times a day. Small errors in the time at which the medications are taken or even how the drugs are taken (before or after a meal) can make a significant difference in the dosage delivered to one's blood and can increase the risk of infection or rejection.

Additionally, Leslie had just moved to a new school after her first transplant, making it more difficult for her to maintain this daily routine, while attempting to blend in with her new classmates. Her transplant coordinator warned her, "You can miss treatments with cystic fibrosis and it might be alright, but with the transplant, the medications need to be taken every day, without fail."Unfortunately, Leslie lapsed and didn't keep up with her treatment protocol. When she next saw her transplant coordinator, the potential consequences of her neglect became all too clear, and she went into a corner of the exam room, pulled her hat over her eyes and began to cry.

It was only a few months after this incident that Leslie went into rejection. First she suffered acute rejection, which was unresponsive to high doses of medications, and then progressed to chronic rejection. She was in and out of the hospital, on oxygen, and having a hard time even climbing the stairs or taking a shower. Leslie did not like to talk about this time in the hospital and only referred to it indirectly. For three or four weeks, she was unsure of whether she would get new lungs. As her lung function declined, Leslie had to consider two alternative realities, one in which she would receive new lungs and one in which she would not and would die.

Illness was isolating and Leslie was often alone in the hospital and spent much of her time with the child life specialist, who was her advocate and link to the other parts of the medical team. Leslie often saw nurses come and go, and she wanted to make sure that they knew her well. The child life specialist helped Leslie design a "Get to know Leslie" quiz for the hospital staff. While the nurses were asking her questions she retorted back with questions from her own quiz.

Leslie was also isolated at home. Her brother was aloof, sometimes uncaring and occasionally abusive. Her mother retreated to work, partly to ensure she could keep her job and benefits, but also out of fear of having to witness Leslie's worsening condition. Leslie had a realistic appreciation of how sick she was but her mother was not there, physically or emotionally, for Leslie to share her fears and emotions. The child life specialist suggested that she write a letter to her mother explaining her feelings, and the nurses gave the letter to Leslie's mom. When Leslie returned to her room, the letter was open but her mother made no attempt to talk about it. Although her mother was not ready to talk to her daughter about her illness, Leslie was thinking about her future. She was hoping for the best but already preparing for the worst.

She first talked to the child life specialist about dying when they were alphabetizing CDs together and listening to music. She mentioned that the song that was playing was one she would like to have played at her funeral. Occasionally, Leslie would speak more nonchalantly about her own passing, using phrases like "when I kick the bucket." But she was thinking about her legacy too, and she began making a video with the child life specialist that captured a day in her life—showing the world how she wanted to be viewed when she was gone, who she was as a person, and not her illness.

The room she was in now was on the same floor as the room where she once had a code blue, when she briefly stopped breathing, became pulseless, and had to be brought back to life. Each moment that she became sicker meant that she rose on the transplant list, just as she inched closer to death. She did receive a second transplant but the memories of that hospital stay are everpresent. As comfortable as she is in the hospital with her clinical team, the distant din of alarms or the overhead speaker can spark painful flashbacks.

Six months later now, following her second transplant, Leslie had banked all of her hope into this second lifesaving intervention—hope that was being tested with this most recent hospitalization, so reminiscent of the complications that led to the rejection of her first transplant. Leslie's nurse walked into her room with a computer, some medications, and a list of questions for her admission paperwork. As the admitting nurse walked through the admission worksheet, she asked her, "What are your concerns for your hospitalization?" This was the question that I wanted to ask since her doctor had told her she had an infection. My mind was ruminating over the worst outcomes that could result from a serious lung infection. Yet, Leslie responded, gently teasing her nurse, "You, of course!" This time, her course would not repeat itself. Leslie recovered quickly from this second bout of RSV, aided with the help of an expensive medication. Despite her recovery, the specter of infection and rejection was never far away. A few months later, I received a text from her mom. Leslie was in the hospital and about to be readmitted. The cycle of fear and uncertainty was repeating itself. This time Leslie had developed a cough and cold during a long awaited trip to Disney World in honor of her sixteenth birthday.

I arrived at Leslie's hospital room just as her team of physicians was speaking with her. Outside the door, as I put on my gown and gloves, I heard a snippet of the conversation. It was laced with the word "rejection." Yet, inside the hospital room, despite requiring oxygen to help her breathe, Leslie seemed to be upbeat and looked better than I had seen her before. Her face was bright and her cheeks full. She looked like she had gained some weight and her hair had grown out, thicker and longer. When her mom left to get Leslie's suitcase from the car and the nurse had finished her intake paperwork, Leslie was excited to tell me about her visit to Disneyworld. She showed me a picture taken on a roller coaster with her friend. Leslie was beaming, arms raised high in the air, looking fearless and embracing the moment, while her friend was reacting just as I would on a roller coaster, crouched into herself, fearful of the descent to come. The trip was less than ideal; she caught a cold and her lung function was declining, but Leslie was ever eager to see the silver lining. Walking through the park was a hassle for her, and she eventually had to use a wheelchair; but with unfettered optimism she claimed, with a beaming smile, "At least in a wheelchair you don't have to wait in line for the rides." The veneer of her smiles couldn't hide her concerns. She was frank with me about the fact that she was not willing to consider a third transplant.

We cannot predict what the future holds for Leslie, but she has come to terms with the permanent frailty of her own life, learning to embrace the moment and bring joy to those around her. When I started medical school, I sought to understand the biological basis of disease and cultivate the skills to diagnose and effectively provide the appropriate intervention for patients' ailments. But Leslie has taught me of the ambiguity in medicine, of how often it is an imperfect science. Despite all our knowledge about the biological underpinnings of cystic fibrosis, we are still able to offer little in terms of cure. Instead,

Leslie's story has demonstrated how often our interventions are incomplete, imperfect and fraught with their own complications. In the process, Leslie taught me the importance of being a physician who is capable of understanding and anticipating the daily struggles that accompany chronic illness, despite the absence of a clear cut intervention.

REVELATIONS

The physician should not treat the disease but the patient who is suffering from it.

— Maimonides

Heartbeats

GALINA GHEIHMAN

They say that doctors are natural storytellers. Perhaps they are not so much storytellers themselves as the conduits by which patients' stories reach a larger audience. For doctors rarely need to work hard to find stories: patients seek their help and tell their stories themselves. So why do I find it so difficult to write this story? Why is it such a struggle to get the words out onto the page, to bring my fingers to the keyboard and spell out what I have seen, heard, and felt? Perhaps because I could never do it justice on the page: I simply could not type so fast or for so long to capture the infinite minuteness of the details I have observed. And not just the millions of pieces that form the scenes I observed and the sounds I heard, but also how all of this was multiplied and amplified and reflected in the feelings, thoughts, and insights that fluttered about me and within me as they happened. I did not know how I felt about becoming a doctor and how this journey would change me. Writing has allowed me to slow my thoughts down, to record how they progressed and changed. Much like an artist exploring scenes and colors and accents on the page to arrive at some new truth, I recognize that reflection, if we allow it to, will often take us into a new place that we may not have intended to go.

Laura was a relatively healthy young woman when she experienced her first grand mal seizure. It started off inconspicuously enough, just another winter evening like any of those previously. She and her husband, Matt, turned in for an early night, as was their custom, with no expectations that anything was amiss. Matt awoke to her thrashing in the bed bedside him and their dog Bella running around the bed and barking up a storm. He was scared and rushed to turn on the lights, revealing a frightening scene. Laura's body was convulsing, her eyes open but rolled back and clearly nonresponsive. He rushed to call 9-1-1 for an ambulance. A few minutes later the seizure was over and Laura awoke, becoming aware of the commotion around her. The dog was still yelping, running back and forth around the bed. Reflecting on the experience sometime later, Matt recalled that Laura had the classic signs of a major epileptic seizure—tonic-clonic contractions, eyes rolling back, foaming at the mouth. He couldn't help it, but for a moment he thought she looked as if she was possessed. His Laura was gone, and a terrible, unknown force had replaced her.

Laura does not recall this story of course. She was unconscious for most of this time; if she was not entirely unconscious, then at least she was not capable of remembering the experience or interacting with others during the seizure. The first thing she remembers is looking around the hospital emergency department and finding herself being wheeled around by Matt in a wheelchair. She remembers her first thought was one of astonished embarrassment, as she gawked at the terrible clothing choice Matt had made in the rush to get her dressed and safely to the hospital. She appreciated his effort, of course, but could not help her gut reaction when she saw the frumpy blouse and decidedly *non-matching* trousers he had managed to pull on. Immediately after this thought, she was intrigued—was this really the first thought she should be having, given the gravity of the situation? And yet it was the thought that came, and it is the memory that has stuck with her since. Fortunately, she responded very well to the medications and has not experienced any grand mal seizures since. She reports no side effects from the medications, but feels "forgetful and needs to make lists," although she is still able to focus and function effectively in her work in administration at a college.

While no one could have predicted the grand mal seizure, once Laura had the diagnosis of epilepsy, she realized there may have been warning signs leading up to it in the preceding years. Three or four years previously, she began to hear an auditory hallucination, what would later be termed her aura—a type of seizure activity that occurs locally in the brain, and often presents as a visual or auditory hallucination. Her aura was the sound of a man talking—a particular man with a deep, smooth voice that would come and go, at first loud in her mind and then softened. This occurred rarely at first, but soon began to increase in frequency. She was not particularly bothered by the hallucination itself, but she was always aware of it occurring, and it would often signal the onset of a subsequent headache. As the voice became increasingly louder and stronger, she became concerned and visited her primary care provider, who attributed the voice to stress and prescribed a sedative and an antidepressant to lift up her mood. Laura was quite taken aback by these suggestions and had absolutely no intention of going on antidepressants or taking strong sedatives. Disappointed that she had been dismissed and did not have an answer to this concerning problem, she tried her best to simply ignore the voice and not allow it to get her down.

While she told her husband about the symptoms, she felt embarrassed and concerned because her grandmother on her father's side had been hospitalized for mental illness. She feared that she too might be experiencing the first signs of mental illness. As such, she was in fact relieved when she was diagnosed with epilepsy and her auditory auras were explained. I would later learn that small auras, increasing in frequency and severity, can signal the onset of a major seizure, much like the one Laura had the night of her diagnosis. Moreover, the auditory hallucinations fit with her eventual diagnosis of left temporal lobe epilepsy—the most common form of adult onset epilepsy and the one most closely tied to auditory hallucinations, because the affected area causing the seizures is located in the auditory center of the temporal lobe in the brain. Since beginning medication, Laura has not experienced another seizure and considers herself to be under excellent control. She will occasionally report hearing the auditory aura of the repeating male voice, but it is much less frequent and certainly less bothersome. She is currently on the newest anti-epileptic drug which is also the safest one for women of child-bearing age.

Following the fateful night in the Emergency Department, and after starting her medications, Laura did not notice any significant changes in her mental or physical health in the early period. However, immediately after being released from hospital, she was not allowed to drive for six months, and it was this restriction that had the greatest impact on her mental health. She was not comfortable relying on others to get her where she needed to go, and suffered from the loss of independence. She felt vulnerable and needy, and resented not being able to care for herself. Those six months she and Matt had to arrange their schedules just so, allowing him to drive her to and pick her up from work as well as taking care of everything that involved needing to drive. This period was perhaps the most trying after her diagnosis, but because she knew it was time-limited, she was able to wait it out and greet her new independence with joy.

When I met my mentor, Dr. Bertill, I learned that she had developed a practice in which she managed women with epilepsy who were either pregnant or in the prime of their reproductive years and interested in becoming pregnant. As a young neurology resident, Dr. Bertill recalled how she had seen many young women with epilepsy. It was the era where new drugs were becoming available, and new formulations developed to minimize side effects helped to regulate and suppress seizures. Importantly for the population of female patients of child-bearing age, the new medications are less apt to cause birth defects than those available previously, meaning that epileptic women have the opportunity to have children in a way that would be safe both for them and for their developing fetus.

These women, however, were not having families, not by choice but because they were afraid. In speaking with her female patients, Dr. Bertill saw that there was a lot of misinformation, and that few patients had a good understanding of what their risks and options were. Many had not even considered the possibility of starting a family. Worse still, some had considered doing so, asking for help from their previous neurologists, only to hear, in a painfully presumptuous and stigmatizing manner, that it would be impossible for them to ever have children. Incensed by the injustice of these stories, and armed with the scientific facts about the true risks of pregnancy and serious congenital malformations for her patients, Dr. Bertill was determined to make it possible for any of her female patients to start a family and live as normal a life as possible. So it was that her career began to take shape. She would work with epileptic females in the clinic, and began leading research projects that would help to continue to build the knowledge that was lacking in this field. As a clinician-scientist, she knew how to pose the right scientific questions by identifying gaps and questions that arose within her own practice; and, in turn, she also could provide patients with the latest and highest quality evidence and information about their choices and the associated risks for their individual condition and circumstances.

According to Dr. Bertill, epilepsy still remains a hidden disease. Those who have it can suffer in silence, and those that manage it well are not proud to disclose this—they fear discrimination by friends, by loved ones and partners, by their work or place of employment, and others. When it comes to pregnancy, these concerns are even greater, but Dr. Bertill does not see managing a pregnancy with epilepsy any differently than managing a pregnant woman with diabetes or hypertension. In all cases of pregnant women who have a chronic illness, they require medications, and they need to strike a balance between managing the benefits of the medications and their risks to try and achieve the best possible outcomes for both mom and baby. The photos of young mothers smiling with infants plastered upon the walls of her office are testament to the career and expertise she has built, and the long lasting relationships she has developed while guiding patients through both some of the most difficult but also the most joyous times in their lives.

Laura was in to see Dr. Bertill primarily to get the "okay" to start trying to conceive with her husband. She was already on the "safest" medications in terms of pregnancy and the risk for major congenital malformations, so there was no need to adjust these and go through the counseling process at that time. However, Dr. Bertill did describe how the dose of these medications might need to increase during pregnancy. Many women find they need to have up to two or three times the dosage of medication by the end of their third trimester.

Laura found out she was pregnant on Christmas Eve and called me two days later. She had not been anticipating a positive test, but in the evening when Matt invited her out to a restaurant with friends, she thought she would check just in case. After all, the party would have alcoholic drinks and in the off chance she was pregnant (though she *highly doubted it* at the time), she would not want to drink that night. She expected to get a negative result and go out to have a good time, but instead she learned the unexpected and joyous news that the pregnancy test was positive! Laura almost could not believe the results, and while Matt was ecstatic as well, the two of them did not quite know what to do with the information. They decided to go to the party anyway, and were relieved to have an excuse to see friends and take this happy but momentous news off their minds. They agreed not to tell anyone at this stage and just go out and have a good time.

The only problem was that a longterm girlfriend of Laura's noticed that she was not drinking that evening, and apparently cornered Matt until he told her the truth about the pregnancy test. Fortunately she did not tell anyone else or question Laura about it, and they were relieved when they were finally able to get home. Laura and Matt did not want to share the news with anyone until the pregnancy had been confirmed, or at least until they completed the first ultrasound. At that point, they would tell their families, and a few weeks later, their friends. They just did not want others to know when there is such a high rate of miscarriage in the first semester—they would not have wanted to share a loss with others should it have happened.

I was so honored that she did, in fact, decide to call, and felt comfortable enough to share this intimate information with me. It was a very special place I found myself in—a new role for me. My job was simply to listen, to be present, to be supportive, and to lend a thoughtful and interested ear.

A few weeks later, I ask Laura how it feels being pregnant. How has she changed physically? How has she changed emotionally? Does she even feel a difference at all? Laura explained that since becoming pregnant she actually does feel very different in terms of her entire sense of her body. She had no idea this would happen, but she describes noticing that she has become much more sensitive in her senses and that her pain tolerance is very low. For example, she accidentally hit her hand and almost could not tolerate the pain, although there was no bruising. Likewise, her sense of smell has sharpened, and she says she is able to smell dinner from the night before when she walks into the kitchen.

Unfortunately, Laura was nauseous almost all the time. She was dizzy and vomiting often, dry-heaving and gagging with little control. Apparently Laura is easily nauseated if travelling long distances by car or train or if she rides a rollercoaster. Now, however, this is worse than she has ever experienced, as it is persistent and constant, and there does not appear to be anything she can do to get relief. She says she can tolerate the dizziness, and even the pain, but the nausea has been completely debilitating, making it almost impossible for her to concentrate or work.

Emotionally, Laura did not report feeling very different. But she did admit that Matt had made some comments about her mood. He suggested, as kindly as possible, that she had been a little bit more snappy than usual lately, and perhaps more emotional, but Laura herself did not see this change. Mostly she was feeling exhausted from all the nausea. She could not keep food down and had even lost weight over the last few weeks as a result. Her sleep was poor too, and trying to concentrate at work while feeling so ill was really wearing her down.

Laura and Matt, at this point, had not started to plan specifically for the arrival of their child, and had not begun making any baby-related purchases. Both of them were very level emotionally—happy about the news, but reserved. Still they did not want to tell friends or family until they had a bit more confirmation, and were in the "safe zone" after 12-15 weeks. Laura stated that she sometimes forgot she was pregnant, but she was sure that seeing the ultrasound in a few weeks time would help the situation seem "more real," and give her the assurance she needed in order to be able to tell her family the good news. They did think it would be safe to discuss some potential baby names. Julia was their top for a girl and Andrew for a boy. Other options, however, included Henry, Peter, or James and, for a girl, Claire or Ada. Some of these represented old names that ran in the family or were variations on other names of close relatives. Neither Laura nor Matt had a particular preference for the sex of their child, but both said they would be glad to know if some evidence was discovered on the first ultrasound.

REVELATIONS

There were other changes that Laura could identify had occurred since she discovered she was pregnant. She found it increasingly difficult to sleep, partly due to nausea and partly due to stress. Since sleep deprivation and stress were triggers for her auras, she worried that this situation might be putting her and the baby at risk. A second source of worry was that neither she nor Matt had family in the area to help. Yet the biggest change Laura noticed, aside from the physical symptoms and the new set of worries, was that the pregnancy had initiated a complete 180-degree turn in their life—including their relationship with one another. They spent almost all their time talking about the child, thinking about the child, and planning for its arrival. It was hard to detach from that focus, and they knew that, at this stage, they were unlikely to go back to the life that they had led together before. But this change also brought about pleasant differences that Laura had not expected. She noticed that Matt had become even more supportive, enthusiastic, and willing to help. Laura often came home from work drained and would fall on the bed to sleep before dinner. In response, Matt graciously took on the job of fixing meals, cleaning the apartment, grocery shopping, and doing anything else that needed to get done. This was a different side of Matt than Laura had seen before, and while she felt very guilty for being ill, she also felt relieved and incredibly loved to have Matt around to help her.

Laura had sought out Dr. Bertill to be her neurologist in Boston, precisely because of her reputation as an expert in the treatment of epilepsy during pregnancy. There are several risks that arise for both the mother and the fetus, should the mother undergo uncontrolled seizure activity during pregnancy, such as miscarriage, premature labor, and still birth. For women themselves, the reemergence of seizures during the pregnancy due to changes in hormone and drug levels can have physical and mental health consequences, challenging women's sense of safety, autonomy, and control. Unfortunately, just at the time when anti-epileptic medication is arguably most important, medication adherence among many women is poor in pregnancy—likely from misinformation about the danger of congenital malformations or unfounded fears that "any drugs during pregnancy are harmful to the fetus." The treatment of epilepsy during pregnancy is a balancing act. The children of women with epilepsy on medications are known to be at slightly increased risk for birth defects. As I learned about these risks, I gained a greater understanding of the importance of Dr. Bertill's work, and how it complemented the care Laura would be receiving from the obstetrician. Both physicians cared for the baby and the mother, but each had different priorities and goals in mind. They would have to work together as both a team and with the patient, in order to achieve an outcome that was best for both mother and child.

One theme that I kept running up against over the course of this experience was that of the "third space," meaning the potential space or distance that exists between the world of our patients (e.g., their beliefs, stories, ideas, and homes) and the world of medicine (e.g., clinic appointments, observations, and our mentors). Between these two is an uncertain, often amorphous, and constantly changing space that we, the medical students, occupy. On a positive note, living in the "third space" offered certain benefits and privileged access to both the world of my patient and the world of medicine. Oftentimes it offered the first step into our patients' lives—and I would leverage the "clinical connection" to ask some difficult questions; but at other times I felt that I was perhaps trespassing beyond the limits of my third space, and encroaching onto property that was the patient's own. All this just as I was starting to grow into my White Coat.

I can't help but feel that I am trespassing into Laura and Matt's lives—it's a very privileged look into an intimate and deeply meaningful and also personal moment in their lives. And, perhaps, "trespassing" is not the right word—after all, Laura has consented to have me learn about her and to shadow with her during the appointment; but I also recognize that I've tumbled deep into very intimate aspects of this couple's life. In a way, we as physicians gain deep access to many aspects of our patients' lives, and yet, in the end, we must recognize that we are only observers and can never be as closely involved as we may want to be. This issue came up for me when I saw Laura in the clinic with Dr. Bertill. Laura was coming in to report the happy news of her pregnancy. I remember thinking ahead about the encounter that morning, and debating whether or not I should wear my White Coat to the clinic. This was less about the physical choice of determining what to wear and, instead, was based on a philosophical choice I was making, i.e., when I walked into the clinic, was I to see myself as a clinician, a future physician-to-be, standing at Dr. Bertill's side and taking notes, observing Laura like any other patient we might see? Or do I switch sides and accompany Laura like a family member might, a support person, someone who does not have the medical expertise but, rather, carries the knowledge of the patient as a person?

I shuffled back and forth between the options, pulling the coat on and off in my mind, and trying to imagine which felt more honest, given this stage of the game. In the end, I didn't wear the coat.

Just a few days later, at Laura's first obstetrics and gynecology (OB/GYN) appointment, I did wear my coat and there wasn't the same kind of agonizing decision that went into it. I hope that the White Coat will not be a barrier to me building genuine, respectful, and equal partnerships with my patients. It might seem frivolous to think about it and to talk about it, but it's not the coat itself that matters—it's the meaning and the symbolism we have imbued it with.

THE SOUL OF A PATIENT

I remember back in our first class in medical school, "Introduction to the Profession," being reminded that as physicians we will be invited to step into all sorts of intimate moments in people lives, and can easily go from asking someone about their day to discussing something intense and deeply personal, such as their struggles with addiction, their sexual history and function, or even how they are dealing with the death of a loved one. We have to be able to step into these roles, but we have to step into them with respect, with acknowledgement of their sacredness, and with humility before the patient. Just like with conversations, we also invade or peer into the private space of our patients' bodies. Sometimes it is just by asking questions, sometimes through physical examinations or other laboratory and imaging tests. With Laura's ultrasound coming up, I can't help but draw the parallels to my feelings of trespassing. Just as I ask questions to glean insights into her life, so too will the ultrasound technician have the chance to peer inside her body. What could be more intimate, private, and personal than looking at the development of her child inside her body—and yet what could be more routine? How is it that we are able to overcome the strangeness and the feelings that these situations raise within us and simply go on with the routineness of the procedures?

I felt lucky to be included in Laura's initial visit to the OB/GYN office, where she would be having a first ultrasound for the baby and, of course, meeting her physicians. It felt almost surreal to be joining Laura and her husband on what was potentially one of the most significant days in their lives. Because Laura was considered a "high-risk mother," given her history of epilepsy and "advanced maternal age," the ultrasound was done at 7 weeks rather than the usual time of between 10 and 13 weeks. It was surprising to me that we were able to see it at all, when, as the ultrasound technician estimated for us, the fetus was only about the size of a blueberry.

For me, the most amazing part of looking at the ultrasound monitor was actually being able to see the little flutter of the fetal heartbeat for the first time. I say "flutter" because it truly looked like a tiny butterfly, no more than a few mm across, that opened and closed its little wings, unfurling them at a remarkably quick pace. I've heard before that hummingbirds can flick their wings as fast as 40 times a second or so, and I was reminded of this remarkable fluttering as I looked on. The baby's heartbeat measured 140 beats per minute. Perfectly healthy.

We zoomed in closer on the monitor, and there the fetus was, curled up like a little pre-historic dinosaur, its head and body and "tail" (we all have what appears to be the remnant of a bony tail at that stage) all part of the normal development in the mother's amniotic sac. It was amazing to realize that in a few short weeks this uterine alien would be recognizable as the little human it would become.

The ultrasound technician said "he" was doing well—and Matthew almost jumped, returning right away with "He? How do you know . . . ?" The technician corrected herself, saying that, actually, she did not know the sex of the baby, and should have called the fetus an "it," but that using "he" was simply easier to say. It's interesting to think about whether this means Matthew was hoping for a boy or not, and this little unconscious slip revealed this preference. I asked him about it later, and he replied that, honestly, the sex did not matter to him, but having the knowledge did, and at the next ultrasound he planned to ask.

The technician printed out a few pictures for Laura and Matthew, and Matthew joked that he should cryptically post an image of the baby on the Internet, perhaps on his Facebook account, without saying anything else. He knew this would drive his mother crazy, since she has been pushing the two of them to have a child for a number of years now, and would expect to be the first to be told the news if they were successful in conceiving. Also during this time, somehow, I don't quite remember how it happened, the baby gained a new nickname—"Spanky." Not quite a girl's name and not quite a boy's name, but that's what made it so perfect. And it stuck! This garnered a round of laughter from everyone, of course, and I fear that, as is the case with the worst of nicknames, it may just continue to live on forever in family lore.

Thinking back on the tiny fetal heart makes me think of the numerous times I have listened to my father's heart. When I was younger, I loved curling up next to my father as he sat on the armchair reading or on the sofa watching the television, and lying my head on his shoulder or further down on his chest. I would press my ear against his heart, and while he sat watching, patting my head and combing his fingers through my hair, I would close my eyes and focus all my attention on the regular *thump-thump, thump-thump* of his heart. I remember this vividly and so fondly, because on one of these occasions I had a significant realization that would affect how I viewed hearts in the future. Somehow, on that one occasion, I realized—and I can't place why it took me so long, but perhaps it was just that I had not *consciously* contemplated these things before as a young kid—that his heart, and my heart, and all the hearts in all the people around me had been beating nonstop since the very first day they came into existence. This was a grand and unparalleled realization, and I remember being not only awed by the mere fact of this truth but by the sheer force of the expansive, fleeting wonder I felt.

I was able to listen to my father's heart and know, reliably, that it had worked continuously for 30 years, and that it would continue to beat for at least as many more years, if not much, much more into the future. Seeing the baby's heart beat, so early in its existence, took me back to this moment of wonder, because it gave me the chance to see it in its earliest form—

only 7 weeks, and already that little heart was pumping away, regular and autonomic, and would continue to do so for the entirety of this little person's life (so little a being it can hardly be called a person!).

After the ultrasound appointment we returned to the clinic waiting room to await our visit with the OB/GYN specialist. As we sat, I noticed that Laura held a piece of paper in her lap with a list of questions to make sure she covered all her bases. I peeked over at the notepad in her lap and saw her questions written in big curly letters, just like one might see on any old to-do list or Post-It note. Unexpectedly, the sentence at the top read *"Am I high risk?"* The loops on the question mark were endearing, as were the curly, gracefully written letters. But somehow the beauty of her penmanship contrasted with the potential threat, the implied worry held in the few words that made up her question. I wondered what it must have felt like for Laura to consider that question, and I also wondered where she found the courage to write it down.

Somewhat unexpectedly, of all the classes I am taking this year, "Medical Ethics and Professionalism" has provided the most insight and relevance to my clinical experience, compared to any of the other medical school classes. Our ethics professor warned us from the beginning that as we learned more and became attuned to these topics, we would begin to see them everywhere. Our topic for the upcoming ethics class was "Abortion." That week we were due to discuss the moral arguments for and against this controversial practice, and, in preparation, we had readings and a short essay response to complete. Since I did not have strong feelings either way, in favor of or against abortion, I was curious to learn what the major arguments on each side have been, and to read true and logical accounts of these arguments, instead of the biased, incomplete, sensationalized information one gets from the media. In short, I gave the topic a lot of thought. As part of the class, we also filled out an anonymous survey. Among numerous questions highlighting particular scenarios and options, I remember being asked "How many people do you personally know who have had an abortion?" I answered "0," reflecting on the fact of how interesting it was that I had comfortably come to conclusions about this topic, and about my own feelings and beliefs on this topic, without ever having had to face it in real life. I had not actually known anyone who had gone through this decision-making process, who had considered or even followed through with this option. On Thursday we had the ethics session—8 students in a small tutorial room with our professor, comfortably and confidently debating our theoretical viewpoints in the safety of the classroom. Here is an excerpt from the conclusion of my assignment for that class, in which I laid out my theoretical stance on abortion and women's right to their own bodies:

In sum, the rights of all patients—pregnant or not—to bodily integrity and informed consent must be respected, "regardless of the impact of that person's choices on others." A woman's autonomous and fully informed choice, made with the interest of both her fetus and herself in mind, should be upheld whenever it is safe to do so.

Little did I know that, just a few days later, I would be staring at my inbox and trying to process the shocking, completely unexpected news that Laura and Matt were considering a termination of their pregnancy, after so many weeks and months of expecting.

Hi Galina,
Unfortunately, we received some pretty bad news about the baby. Last Monday, the test results came back positive for Down syndrome. This has left us with an agonizing and ethical decision to make - whether or not to continue the pregnancy. We'll make a final decision

once the results are back. They are also testing to see if this is something I carry or that will affect any future pregnancies, should Matt and I want to try for another baby down the line.

Perhaps we can meet to discuss in a few weeks. It's still quite painful to speak about and I'm barely holding it together as is. By that time, our decision will be made as well and I'll be, hopefully, in a much better emotional state by then. Sorry to delay meeting; I do want to meet, I just can't right now.

Laura

I remember thinking at the time, "Only last week I did not know anyone who had had an abortion, and here was the very patient I was following preparing herself to undergo one." Before I heard from her on Monday, I had already begun work on the following week's Ethics assignment. This session focused on the ethics of genetic testing. Again we were presented with cases and readings, arguing for and against early screening and what consequences it might have. Of course I thought about Laura as I read through them—after all, I had been able to witness the process of genetic counseling in person, and to have seen Laura and Matt elect to take these tests. But, somehow, the consequences had not been explicit to me at that time—perhaps it had not been to any of us, as we were always inclined to think only optimistic thoughts about the outcome of the pregnancy.

I thought this would be a story about a baby, about pregnancy, birth, new life. What I couldn't have anticipated was that it would also be a story about death. Perhaps I should have expected this—for you cannot have life without death. As Irvin D. Yalom writes in his intelligent, empathetic autobiography about death experiences, looking at death can be like "staring at the sun." We're safer to explore it indirectly or at a tangential angle rather than head on; that is often all that we can handle.

It was not long after the first email from Laura that I received the following devastating news: Laura and Matt had decided to terminate the pregnancy at this time. In no way was I prepared for this news, and my first reaction was deep and disturbed. I was hurt, even shocked by the news, and I could only imagine what they must have been going through. How difficult the discussions they had and the process of making a final choice must have been. It would be weeks before we spoke again.

Hi Galina,

Thank you for your kind voicemail last night. I was on the other line with my mom talking about everything. Matt and I have decided to end the pregnancy, so I'm in the middle of trying to make the arrangements to do so, as well as securing some counseling/therapy for us. I'll be in touch over the next few weeks. Thank you for keeping us in your thoughts.

Laura

After receiving the news from Laura that she planned to terminate her pregnancy, I walked around stunned, not knowing how to feel or how to react to the situation. I was strongly affected—but what exact emotions was I feeling? This I could not say. I struggled to understand, and I was afraid at first to ask for help. It's not that I did not want to speak with someone. It's that I was not yet ready to speak. I felt ashamed somehow, and was grieving for the fact that this situation had come to be this way. Of course, no one would have wanted this, nor could anyone have predicted it, but, nevertheless, I felt we had been tricked, swindled, taken advantage of and left to pick up the broken pieces. It took a while for me to realize that what I was experiencing was grief, and that what I was dealing with was, in every essence, my first death.

I feel like I am holding onto a huge secret—and not just any secret, but a terrible secret. A secret that I am afraid to speak to others about, one I'm practically ashamed to speak about. I'm not sure why that is, given that, on the surface, I think I am alright with genetic testing and even abortion; and yet I feel that there is so much involved in this process that it's almost impossible to know exactly what my true feelings are, and how they are intermixed with, and separate from, my thoughts or ideas on the issue. Should our feelings not be consistent with our thoughts or actions?

In the moments after first learning about Laura's results, I have to say one of the strongest feelings I had was a real sense of mourning. It was a loss, after all, and I could not help but wonder how Laura and Matt were feeling, and what this would mean for their relationship, for their future, and for what we were experiencing together. The termination, aborted not only the child but the dreams, feelings, hopes, and experiences it represented and engendered.

Just prior to learning the diagnosis from Laura, my thoughts regarding these topics before this event seemed to be relatively straightforward. I believed that women should be informed about their choices, but ultimately it was up to them to make a decision about whether they have the resources, emotional wherewithal, and ability to carry and care for, and, ultimately, parent the child. I do not think it is our place to judge whether a woman chooses to continue to carry the child, or, on the other hand, to terminate the pregnancy. Laura and I had even discussed her thoughts on the topic before—and termination and abortion was not totally off the table; but, each time, she said only, "We'll cross that bridge if we ever get to it." At the same time, I got a sense that she and Matt would not be prepared to raise a child that they anticipated would have a significant disability; it was just not something they felt they had the ability to do at this point. So whether Laura somehow implied it or whether I assumed it because of my own biases, I cannot say their decision came as a surprise.

I spent almost two weeks in silence, trying to process and understand my emotions. When I finally got to talking, I decided to speak first with my father, whom I have often used as a guide and mentor when faced with circumstances that challenged me to think and feel in new ways. I phoned him and asked whether he would be willing to simply listen, not necessarily to advise me or answer my questions, but simply provide an avenue to get my thoughts out and a bouncing-board to help me analyze them.

I also didn't know what to do. Should I email her, should I call her, should I say that I got her email, or whatever? So this was all two or three weeks ago, and I tried to . . . I mean I had a lot of my own feelings, but I tried to just put those aside realizing this was not about me, it was about her. So I just called and left a message, saying, "I really appreciate that you emailed me, thank you for telling me this information. I really wish the news was different and that you weren't facing this difficult situation. I know that you and your husband need time and space, so no pressure to call me back, but if you have questions, or I can help . . . please call me."

Some people in my class will say, "I know a child with Down's and he is really happy. He really enjoys his life and he is not suffering. And his family also really enjoys their life and is very happy. Having this child has taught them what is important in life. Everyone's fine . . . and based on that . . . I think that *that* life is worth living." BUT, on the other hand, we know that most people who find out that their child has Down syndrome (DS) during the early fetal genetic testing will choose abortion.

So, I'm very confused; well, actually, maybe I'm not confused. When it comes down to it, it's about *parental expectations.* They want their child to be a certain way—right—and a child with DS may not meet the conditions they are expecting when having a child. But I guess that begs the question "Where do you draw the line?" This is the responsibility of the parent—

to parent the child that they bring into the world, and help them to reach their potential, whatever that may be, but not to put on unnecessary expectations. The same as my child may not be an athlete, or may not be smart at math, or something else, so where is that line? Does it apply for Down syndrome? With Down's, people typically think of the intellectual disabilities, but there are a lot of other potential issues, such as cardiac problems that may come with it. My father reminded me that many people will make many different choices. As a physician, you don't need to decide for *all the people*. And these people, they are your patients. They are not breaking the law. And they do what society allows them to do. So your responsibility is to support them, without passing your own judgments. But, if you will have to make your own choice, you will have your own considerations.

My father has an analogy that he often uses to describe emotions, when he is advising my sister or me. He says that emotions are like a "wave," and one must learn to surf on them. Our consciousness is only the surface waters, and below that is a much deeper, more complex subconscious. Just like when we swim in the oceans, we sometimes see waves coming and we sometimes do not, but either way there is nothing we can do to stop that wave, as it propagates up and along the surface. We have a few options: we can try and surf the wave, coasting along to see where it will take us, or, if we are not careful, it may overtake and overwhelm us. The small waves may just bump us along in an uncomfortable way or direct us down a different trajectory, but the biggest ones may be tumultuous and threatening, and can even pull us under. So just like with waves, we can allow our emotions to overwhelm us (literally crashing over), or we can try and pull ourselves to their surface, acknowledging and feeling them go by, and yet remaining with our head above water. Sometimes, if the emotion hits us just at the right time and place—and we are ready for it—we may even stand up and surf along. It's these moments where the emotion can truly drive us and take us somewhere new, further than we've ever been or we ever thought we could go.

I'm embarrassed to admit I did not see the tsunami that hit me when the news came. I was able to process the results intellectually, but what I had not been prepared for were the feelings that would arise as a result of this knowledge. Once they began—much of them within the negative realm of shame, guilt, and fear on my own part and on the part of my patient—it was much easier to bury them than to try and expose them for examination. These are still stigmatized topics in many ways, and I did not feel that I had a strong enough feeling, either way, to be able to seek advice. I worried at that time about falling to pieces, and knew that what I needed was not someone who could discuss the ethics, or practices, or technicalities of the procedure, but just someone who could provide support—personal support—to me. I knew I had to do that hard work, that I could not keep denying what I felt if I wanted to be able to explore this with Laura in a helpful and supportive way. I could not be battling my own unstable emotions while also trying to be a source and foundation of stability of support for her, should she need it. I knew that by exploring and coming to terms with my feelings, whatever they were, would at least allow me to be open and receptive to hearing her needs and responding to them.

Without realizing it, this was my first introduction to a key component of my professional duty as a physician: balancing one's own emotions and opinions for what should be done, and one's response to a situation against the needs, thoughts, and feelings of our patients. It is all too easy to default to one's own beliefs, but the trick in becoming an open, caring clinician is to be able to solicit and support your patient's needs at the time of their care, rather than your own. This is not to say that you cannot *have* feelings in response to a patient's situation. Feelings are a natural part of us and will come and go whether we want them or not. Our role is to learn to manage our emotions so that we can, instead, focus on the patient. And I should emphasize that managing does not mean ignoring or putting them aside. In fact, it takes real skill, focus, attention, and even mindfulness of sorts to be able to tune into these emotions and to get a reading on one's own body and mind, for this can inform our approach to the patient. In other words, it is in our own and our patient's best interests that we allow our emotions to push us forward and propel us across the waters, rather than overwhelming and drowning our efforts. But doing so takes skill and practice—and not being afraid to get up on the board and face the approaching waters.

I was afraid to speak, afraid to think, and afraid to feel. And while I am not proud that this wave had engulfed me, churning me around and nearly drowning me within it, as my father always said, even that wave passed, eventually. And as I regained my steadiness, swam back out and pulled my head above water, I finally began to see that the receding wave was not actually as big, not actually as scary, and not actually as dangerous as I had feared when stuck within it. I regained my baseline, and only from this safer spot was I ready to begin discussing and exploring what had happened to Laura, and, in response, what had happened to me.

There is a real intimacy and closeness that comes from getting to know someone within the context of medical inquiry. I might go so far as to call it an "accelerated acquaintanceship," where within moments of getting to know someone for the first time we may find ourselves asking deeply personal questions, and, in many cases, even examining their body. This unparalleled speed of intimacy is part and parcel of the medical tradition. It works not because both parties (the patient and the physician) are comfortable with these events necessarily, but rather because we both have our expectations for what "social script" will be followed in the visit. These social norms allow the patient and the physician to get close, fast—hopefully without the patient feeling exposed or losing trust in the physician. As a relationship builds over time (as I hope it does between most patients and physicians seeing one another longitudinally), the genuine intimacy of friendship becomes on par with that initial clinical, strictly professional, intimacy.

There is a great power that comes with putting on the White Coat and taking on the position of the physician. We can ask questions I wouldn't even dream of asking some of my close friends, for risk of offending them, or being perceived as prying into business that is not my own. Yet, we ask patients questions of this nature all the time. We ask if they smoke and drink, and how much. We ask if they've used recreational drugs (now or in the past). We ask how many sexual partners they have had (and if and how they use protection), and we even expect patients to recall their family histories and the dates and causes of death of some of their most intimate relations. Most surprisingly is that patients answer, and they answer promptly, wholeheartedly, and, for the most part, honestly.

White Coat or not, to some extent I still presented myself to Laura as a member of the medical team, and she in turn presented herself as a patient. Under these mutual terms, and at this stage of my development as a physician, I was thus granted permission to question, probe, and examine more deeply some of the issues and topics that might have been off limits in any other type of interaction. But I also realized that knowing someone's most personal "secrets," or looking at their body or deeply within it, is not sufficient to get to know who someone is. Perhaps in medicine we are most at risk of making this false assumption. Because we know the medical history, we presume we know the person, but in fact we know only the slice of their lives that either presents to us in the physical examination or the clinical findings, or that they consent to sharing during the interview. But just as two friends having coffee will discuss family, friends, work, and daily struggles, but seldom get to a history of medications, medical complications, or personal health goals and practices, so too will we as physicians hear great detail of the latter aspects with little time for discussion and exploration of the former.

We *do* learn a lot about our patients (and about their *medical conditions*), but we would be fooling ourselves if we thought that we know everything about them. In fact, it became exceedingly clear over the course of the year that I had now gotten to know Laura much better than my mentor ever had the chance to do. Dr. Bertill had seen her multiple times, yes, but all within the medical context. And Laura's friends and colleagues had seen her personal and social life. But where did that leave me? Straddling somewhere halfway in between, a third perspective that was not-quite-physician and not-quite-friend. Speaking with Dr. Bertill about Laura really brought this realization home. At the end of one conversation, after having explained to Dr. Bertill the discussion I had had with Laura earlier, and her thoughts and feeling surrounding an issue, Dr. Bertill paused, looked around thoughtfully, and then commented: "You know, you are lucky to be getting to know Laura right now as well as you have. In my role in the office, I try to get to know patients well, but I have never gotten to know them or their lives as well as you have with Laura." I hope to fight against this state of affairs through my training and into my practice. It is not necessary for her to know absolutely everything about each patient, but what a shame that our health system does not value physicians building deeper relationships that take perhaps that most valuable of all commodities—time.

Dr. Bertill does not see "the truth between the visits," just as we do not see characters' lives between scenes in a play. But imagine how much richer of an experience we could have, how much deeper and more nuanced an understanding we could have, of the motivations and emotions, or drives and behaviors, or barriers and opportunities, of the characters, if only we could sneak a peek behind the curtains at the working of the backstage world.

In the same way, we do not see the entirety of our patients, but only the "scenes" that play out in the spotlight of the clinic. Often we are left guessing about what has happened in between. Did the patient understand what we discussed? Are they following the plan at home? What barriers are keeping them from following the plan? What motivators or practices have they put in place to be adherents to the plan? Where have we misunderstood or miscalculated, and where can we intervene? My wisest insights along this journey have come from my patient herself. As Laura told me shortly after she learned the results of her genetic screening test, after days of agony trying to understand what had happened with Matt, to come to terms with it, and to make a decision about how they would move forward, "Now that you have seen it, you will know what a test result means for a patient. The hours, and even days, of feeling and thinking that go into processing it. You will know what it means for your patients, because you have seen what it means for us, and for me."

Laura was right, as she so often was. I would not forget this—not just the specifics of her situation, but the greater lesson that, as physicians, we cannot just take what we hear and see in clinic as the end-all and be-all of the patient's experience. Even though our patients' lives may not seem directly related to their medical conditions at first, how could they possibly not be? Our body and our health are not specialized compartments of ourselves that we can isolate and deal with separately from every other component that makes up our lives. Fortunately or unfortunately, this is not the case. Perhaps it is easier to treat our bodies like automobiles coming in for an oil check and a mechanical fix here and there, but even this analogy fails, for the state of the car will depend not only on its mechanics and physical form, but on the experience it has had on the road. Have the roads been rough or smooth? Is the oil that fuels it regular or refined? How often is it driven? And does it get a change of tires in the winter to prevent damage?

So too with our bodies and with our health. We carry our health with us each day, and what we experience in our lives reflects upon it. As physicians, it is our responsibility to probe further, to know our patients intimately, and to open the curtains shielding their true selves from our eyes.

Hi Galina,

Matt and I are doing much better. It's still difficult, but I can now talk about it without crying, which is a huge improvement. I'm back at work as well which helps keep my mind of off things a bit. I have an appointment with Dr. Bertill coming up - are you able to attend that? If not, I can see if she can reschedule. I hope you had a good spring break and that you were able to enjoy your time off!

Laura

One of the important pieces of this experience has been the process of developing a relationship over time with my clinical mentor, Dr. Bertill. I have to admit that when I first met Dr. Bertill I was a bit worried about what the experience would be like, and whether the two of us would "hit it off" or not. I was hoping to have a very warm, helpful, and incredibly dedicated mentor who would have time to teach me, explore with me, offer suggestions, and connect me with others. Instead, I found that she too had little idea about what we *should* be doing, as it was her first year as mentor with the program. So the two of us were discovering this for ourselves in real time, and the boundaries and settings and expectations were malleable, waiting to be set by us.

THE SOUL OF A PATIENT

Dr. Bertill gives off a sense of ultimate competence. She is professional, intelligent, articulate, and confident. She holds and possesses authority, but in a respectful, non-demanding way. You know you are dealing with an expert, with a scientist, someone who has worked hard to get to the place they have reached today, and expects to be treated with the respect she deserves. It was interesting getting to know her at first, because I almost felt that she was a bit cold, emotionally, or at least not as friendly and warm as I might have expected for a female physician whose main clientele and population of interest is women in their child-bearing years. I remember meeting her and feeling some pressure and discomfort, and not being sure whether to be more open or closed in my relationship. I had questions I wanted to ask but I was afraid to demonstrate weakness or lack of knowledge, and a little afraid to set myself up for criticism, given the impression I got from her, that she was very rigorous, very organized, and did not really have any time to waste, not for a first year medical student with stupid questions, nor for anything else.

I remember looking around her office and trying to reconcile a photograph I saw on the wall with the woman who was sitting in front of me. On the photograph was Dr. Bertill, pictured with one of her patients and that woman's young, healthy, and intact child. All three were smiling widely and looking ever so glad to be there together. Dr. Bertill's hair was longer in the photograph and she looked a bit younger, perhaps, but it could not have been too many years ago. Now, it wasn't that she did not smile with me, but it did take a little bit of a while for us to warm up to each other, I guess. I left the first day feeling worried about how this entire course would go. Dr. Bertill had not prepared a patient for me (as I had expected she would), and stated that we would find one together at the next clinic session that I would be able to attend. I thought this was quite unorganized and somewhat unprepared of her, and worried about having to "do everything myself." And it turned out at later sessions that, yes, indeed, the project would require me to take more initiative and to determine independently how many times I would meet with Laura, how many times I would meet with Dr. Bertill, and how I would communicate with both of them between and around sessions.

I never saw Laura in a hospital gown. I never saw her carrying an IV pole, lying in bed, or being struck down by her illness. In so many ways, she was not your typical patient, or at least not the one I imagined when I got signed up to participate in this project. And while Laura did not present as a patient in her appearance—and one might even argue was never acutely physically ill in the time that I knew her—her story still contains all the elements that one associates with the illness narrative. IV pole or not, Laura still experienced the vulnerability, the uncertainty, and the loss of privacy that comes with becoming a patient.

So what qualities *do* identify the patient, if it is not a hospital gown or other such physically obvious stigmata? What I have learned from Laura is that being a patient means being vulnerable—being threatened by something from within or outside of oneself. But perhaps the greater lesson Laura demonstrated was that being vulnerable did not mean that one was helpless, or that one had to be passive. In fact, Laura, as a patient, was the perfect example of what one could do to be active in one's illness, to demand care, to be proactive and engaged, educated, and self-directed. Laura was really the first patient I met who had done reading about her condition on the Internet. She was an exemplary model for the engaged and activated patient who took responsibility for his or her own care. First, Laura had researched all her providers and made a choice about which physician to visit based on online recommendations and expertise. Her "very generous" health insurance plan, as she called it, allowed her to visit almost any provider within

Boston, and, as she said it, she felt lucky that she could see top-tier providers at world class hospitals. She had the confidence to seek the best care for herself, and also the competence to navigate the health system and to find and demand excellence for herself. I have to admit I was quite impressed by this, and the fact that Laura did not allow her illness to possess or over-whelm her.

At the beginning of our relationship, I wondered whether she did think about it much of the time, and was surprised to find it was not at all at the top of her mind. It also helped me realize that I was, perhaps, much more of an anxious person-ality than Laura was. Sometimes I worried about even asking a question or bringing up a topic that might be worrisome or painful for her. For example, I worried about asking her how she felt her epilepsy might affect the pregnancy or whether she was worried about the risks of side effects of her medications? But when I did ask these questions, Laura was rarely fazed. And unlike so many of the patients I had seen before, she re-ferred to the data she had read or the information the doctor had provided as the justification for why she was not con-cerned and did not feel she had to be concerned.

Our conversation began with me asking Laura what, for her, were the key important qualities a physician should possess. She listed many important ones like knowledge, com-petence, compassion, and trustworthiness. But when it came down to it, she said the physician should ultimately "be some-one who you feel comfortable interacting with and speaking with." She thought no one should ever feel uncomfortable with his or her physician and, moreover, that if a person felt that way, he or she should end the relationship and find another provider. She said it very matter-of-factly, and it struck me, perhaps because I understood that in the case of many other patients, going to *any provider* was already a privilege they felt grateful for, and many would not think twice about changing providers or trying to find someone who seemed "better" or more "patient-centered." They simply did not see this as an option they were entitled to. It takes a certain kind of savvy and a level of education and self-respect to be able to do so.

Laura and Matt invited me for a visit in their home on the second weekend in May, perfectly timed to coincide with the late arrival of spring in Boston this year. To visit Laura and Matt at home, I had to take the subway and the bus to travel closer to their neighborhood, in a suburb outside of Boston. When I stepped out of the train on the other side, the difference couldn't have been more palpable. Far from the city and its influences, I felt that the suburb offered a safe haven, with fresh air to breathe, colorful flowers to smell and admire, and seemingly more relaxed individuals going about their day. The pace of activity seemed to slow down here, and the hum of the city—streetcars rolling by, honking horns, and squealing buses stopping abruptly at the curb—was no more. It was a perfectly sunny day, and on the Sunday afternoon that I visited, several young families with their children were outdoors near Laura's home, taking advantage of the early signs of the impending summer.

Laura pulled the door to let me in, and what greeted me was not a brightly lit open hallway, as I had expected, peeking through the little window in the door, but, instead, an incredibly large, friendly dog! I knew that Laura and Matt had a pet, Bullseye, but I had not realized just how large he was. He jumped up a little as I tried to move inside, and placed his front paws on my collapsing knees. I tried to back up but the space was limited, and Bullseye was intent on greeting me in the friendliest way that he knew how.

Laura invited me for an afternoon visit. I brought along some chocolate for us to share, and Laura had lovingly put out a mixed platter with sliced baguette, home-made green bean and avocado paste, and a fresh slice of brie she had picked up from the local grocery store that morning. It was quite the spread, given that she'd warned me she would not be cooking. It was an unexpected treat, and it nailed home for me that today's meeting was going to mean much more than one of our regular meetings. We would not only be sharing histories, sharing opinions, or sharing stories, but we would be sharing that most fundamental of activities that can bring two people closer: we would be sharing a meal.

Here, in her home, there was no need to debrief or to reflect with specificity about the experience—it was just time we had both committed to share. There was little agenda other than to enjoy an evening together, and I think this freed up the space for a greater diversity of conversation topics. In fact, it really was a conversation more than an interview, and perhaps because we were able to get away from topics of health and healthcare, Laura became more animated, lively, and enthusiastic. I too became more engaged with the discussion, as Laura asked me questions about my personal life, how school was going, and what my interests were for the future. Although Laura was always very friendly and open, our conversations, at least in some part, always felt a bit sterile and controlled; perhaps being in the hospital setting when we had them contributed to this. At home she was open, free, allowed to say and ask what she wished. It was a different side of Laura than I had seen before, and it made me realize how much of our patients we can miss in clinic. The home visit, in this sense, was a real treasure for getting to know Laura on her own terms.

Just as we cannot write the patient note until we have completed the entire history and physical examination, so, too, we cannot know the full story until we have come to its end. In my last meeting of the year with Dr. Bertill, we reflected on how this experience had been for each of us over the course of the last year—the ups and downs in treating and spending time with Laura—and both the expected and unexpected outcomes of participating in this course. As Dr. Bertill expressed it: "You can plan and plan to address the science of the disease as you now know it . . . and yet you must expect the unexpected."

Dr. Bertill believed that taking on a professional role was part of her responsibility to the patient. She wanted to demonstrate expertise, confidence, and competence, so that the patients, too, could feel they could rely on her as a physician— that they would have confidence in her and feel their care was in the right hands. It is hard to instill confidence if you are susceptible to your emotions, however; and, so, perhaps these two qualities are two opposite sides of the same coin, which we must learn to balance. As Dr. Bertill said, "Remember, when you sit with your patient and listen to them, you must listen wholeheartedly, but you must also remember you have another room full of patients waiting for your help." Her point, I believe, was that you absolutely *had* to be a good doctor for your patient, but, even more so, you had to be a good doctor for *all* your patients. The only way to accomplish this fairly was to recognize that your time must be split among them fairly; you cannot let yourself empathize so strongly with each patient that it leaves you empty and incapable of helping the next one.

I think this balance, between sympathizing and holding my emotions back, is one of the lessons that has been hardest for me, and that I anticipate I will continue to struggle with throughout my training. I learned over this experience that sometimes our own emotions in a situation can be unpredictable—sometimes they are less than we might have expected, sometimes more. As we wrapped up our final meeting, I asked Dr. Bertill if she had any final word of wisdom to impart. She said, "What I've learned is that every patient is so different. You cannot predict a patient's response, especially when they are faced with a difficult medical situation that is scary or concerning to them. Some of the women in my clinic come in and they are . . . just scared and worried. And others are cool as a cu-

cumber, throughout it all. But all of them are our patients. And our role is to be sensitive to their specific needs, whatever they may be."

Be sensitive, be helpful, and tend to the needs your patients express. It is both the simplest and most difficult thing—and it is what we as physicians must learn to do.

***

"Long is the road from conception to completion." — Moliere

Month One

Month one is point zero; it is where everything begins. At conception, the female egg is fertilized, and it begins to grow as it travels down the fallopian tubes. A watertight sac grows around it, as if safely enwrapping the delicate ovum in its arms. The amniotic sac will continue to cushion the embryo as it grows. One cell miraculously proliferates into two, then four, then eight, and onwards exponentially based upon the instructions borne out of the uniting of mother and father's DNA. At this time, the embryo's first partner—the placenta—begins to develop as well. For many months, it will serve as a cardiovascular system, liver, gut, and lungs, transferring nutrients and oxygen from the mother in and carrying wastes out. By the end of the first month, the fetus is only about the length of a grain of rice. Circulation has only just begun its infinite loop, and blood cells are forming for the first time. A primitive face—with large circles where the eyes will grow and the first etchings of a mouth, jaw, and throat—is recognizable by the end of this first month. Is it not remarkable that our face, the very means by which we greet others, recognize others, and come to know them—the very thing that identifies us as human beings—is also the first to develop?

Month Two

In month two, the face continues to develop—after all we were still missing the ears, eyes, and nose in month one. Small projections begin to bud off the body as well, growing outwards in four symmetric directions. These early forms will soon become limbs, with delicate elaborations beginning to mark out fingers and toes. Substantial changes on the outside are paired with an intricate maze of events on the inside of the fetus, as neural and gastrointestinal tubes swell, encircle, twist and turn. The head is largest early on but bone is soon laid down in place of cartilage and gives the body its increasing weight. By the end of the second month, the embryo grows to about an inch in size, no larger than a berry. It is at this point that it ceases to be an embryo and earns the name of fetus. The development of ears at this time may seem unimportant, and is often forgotten in the midst of excitement about the development of vital internal organs or other complex external structures like the eyes. And yet the ears are fundamental. It is with the ears that we listen. It is with our ears that we hear our patients' stories.

Month Three

The final month of the first trimester in many ways encapsulates the entire phenomenon from conception to delivery. By the end of month three, all of the rudimentary elements of the baby are fully formed; its anatomy and organ systems are in place. From here, they will continue to grow and mature; beginning to adopt the complex functions they will serve in the infant after birth. The baby at this time is only about the length of a pencil and weighs no more than an ounce, and yet the circulatory system has begun to flow, the kidneys to filter, and the liver to churn out bile. It is as if the organs one by one come online, slowly taking over the functions the placenta has so willingly served during the first critical weeks of development. Sexual development is also complete—if you look for it, you may even discern the gender of the baby on ultrasound. Precarious as pregnancy itself then, Month three and the end of the first trimester is truly an inflection point. After this stage, the baby's most critical developmental phase is primarily complete, and the rate of miscarriage drops accordingly.

Month Four

At the start of the second trimester, the baby's heartbeat becomes clearly audible, and can be detected using a sound wave instrument called a Doppler. The heart begins its formation many weeks before now but as with other parts of our development, there are several stages of transformation and maturation until it takes its final shape. Mothers-to-be will often have their first ultrasound in this period; it is a time of new beginnings, of introductions, of new relationships. We greet baby, and he or she may greet us back: eyelids, eyebrows, eyelashes, nose, and mouth are now fully formed and many parents claim to see facial expressions on ultrasound, or at the very least junior yawning and sucking his or her thumb. With new beginnings comes new growth, and by the end of the fourth month, the baby almost doubles in length, stretching from the tip of its head down to its finely formed fingers and toes.

Month Five

In month five, the events of development take on a quicker pace. The baby is developing muscles and beginning to exercise them— mothers often clue into this process as they feel the first exciting kicks from deep within their belly. It is a time of joy and unconscious expectations—if Junior is a strong kicker, his parents may joke that he will be a soccer player or she will be a dancer. Already ideas and hopes are emerging, growing and maturing along with the child who will be asked to fulfill them. Unexpectedly perhaps, the baby also begins to grow hair during this interval. At the time, its shoulders, back, and parts of the face and head will be covered with lanugo, a soft, fine layer of hair. This will remain until the first week of life; it is one of the earliest of many protective layers we grow and then must shed as we age and mature, growing stronger.

Month Six

Some have called month six the threshold point. By the end of the second trimester, the baby is making its presence known. On average, almost a foot in length and two to three pounds in weight, it moves from side to side, jerks, hiccups, and may respond to sounds with a quickening of its heartbeat. Its eyelids may part and the eyes open, as if the child were surveying its otherworldly, underwater scene. It's a threshold because up until this point the baby has relied entirely upon the mother's body for nutrients, protection, and survival. With some support however, it may be able to live outside the womb. It's fitting then that the child's finger and toe prints become visible, marking an identity of its own.

Month Seven

Month seven marks the start of the third and final trimester of development. It is a joyous time—the final growth phase of the baby will soon begin. In all likelihood, even babies born prematurely during this time are likely to survive. As the baby grows and matures, it will begin to lay down reserves of body fat for the future as well as begin building muscles and other energy stores. This is a slow process, with many metabolic changes occurring over time. An investment for the preservation of the self; an investment for the future. A new balance is struck as the baby grows in size within the womb, causing the amniotic fluid to recede. Not yet complete in its sensory development entirely, the fetus can nevertheless respond to important, rudimentary stimuli, including pain, light, and sounds. We believe the baby may soon be capable of hearing mother's voice, perhaps beginning to build its first and most important relationship at this time.

Month Eight

In the penultimate month of development, the fetus continues to grow, gaining strength in its muscle and bones and building reserves of fat for the long term. Development of the brain continues at an increasing pace, with some of the fundamental, early circuits being laid down and consolidated. While still within its amniotic haven, the child can now see and hear; its auditory and visual systems scanning the environment and learning to respond. The baby's organ systems should be fully developed by the end of the eighth month, except for the lungs, which often do not complete maturation until after birth. Connected via the placenta, the baby still feeds and breathes through the mother. But the organ systems are revving up to begin their own independent life—symbolically and physically liberated with the cutting of the umbilical cord. Perhaps ironically, it is through this process of gaining independence that the parts of the body become a whole—they do not act alone, but are all necessary components of an intricate system. Systems that both enable and constrain.

Month Nine

The ninth and final month of pregnancy marks both a new beginning and an end. It is the final stage, and yet it is also the origin of something entirely and unknowingly new. In these last short weeks, the baby grows and grows, until there is hardly room left for it within. It moves less due to the space constraints—although he or she will take one last flip to prepare for labor and delivery. What final parts must be in place? What final connections and circuits must be wired to begin? Rather than embellish with complexity, it is the rudimentary circuits that are connected, and the baby's reflexes are complete: the fetus can blink, respond to lights, sounds, and touch, grasp tightly, and turn its head in response to noise. The baby has never been more ready to greet the world! It has reached its final weight; it has reached its final length. It is ready to end, and in so ending, ever more ready to begin. The end of an era, and the origin of a new life.

Sacrifices

ITHAN PELTAN

Everyone who is born holds dual citizenship in the kingdom of the well and in the kingdom of the sick. Although we all prefer to use only the good passport, sooner or later each of us is obliged, at least for a spell, to identify ourselves as citizens of that other place.

— Susan Sontag

It is not difficult to imagine the flat and bleak and barren terrain of the country that Susan Sontag discovered during her battle with cancer. As a first-year medical student, I believed that nobody would dwell in the kingdom of the sick longer than necessary. This conviction was soon shaken by my exposure to Vinnie Terrazo. Our time together, a series of long afternoons spent talking in cold exam rooms throughout my first year of medical school, forced me to confront a disturbing question: What happens when a person surrenders his passport to the kingdom of the well? This wasn't someone with terminal illness, but rather, someone who could have enjoyed the sunny fields of health by objective medical criteria. Vinnie seemed to have voluntarily chosen permanent residency in the kingdom of the sick. But why?

Vinnie was 65 years-old and suffered from a long list of diseases, including diabetes, an inflammatory condition affecting his digestive system called Crohn's disease, heart disease, and a clotting disorder. Dr. Aronson had cared for Vinnie and coordinated his extensive consumption of medical services for many years. Although he was not a healthy man, Vinnie was as well as could be expected. His cardiac stress tests were clear, his blood sugar control nearly ideal, and both his clotting and digestive disorders were under the best control that medicine could offer. Modern medicine had provided Vinnie with relief from his multiple chronic diseases.

Yet, Vinnie radiated depression. **A**n afternoon with him always left me sad and his tone of perpetual complaint conveyed exhaustion brought on by a battle against overwhelming odds. He was an obese, shabby bald man with a bull neck. He lived alone in the same house in the working-class neighborhood where he grew up with his Italian-American family. Though perpetually shocked at the passage of the years, he wore a talking watch that announced the turn of the hour all day and all night. Vinnie described himself as a life-long "loner" but thrived on social relationships. He was happiest on days filled with human contact, yet the sustenance he derived did not originate in the simple pleasure of the interaction. The first time I asked Vinnie a standard question of the medical interview, "What makes you feel healthier?" he told me that "having someone (a woman) in my life" was the single thing most likely to make him feel better, not about himself as a person, but about his *health*.

The saga of Vinnie's family life, described from his point of view, illustrates the structure of his relationships and the problems he had maintaining them. His teenage habit of trolling for vulnerable women willing to trade companionship for a ride in his brightly-painted muscle cars began a pattern of barter-based and even predatory sexual relationships that continued throughout his life. Vinnie met his first wife Maria during a vacation to Italy shortly after high school, where a fake marriage to procure her a green card turned sour when the priest sent the marriage certificate to the central registry. After two years of living together, the relationship ended when Maria's real husband returned from the Italian Army. Vinnie eventually obtained a civil divorce, but only after a long effort to have the marriage annulled by the Catholic Church failed. Vinnie's inability to blame himself for anything explains why the annulment merited so much effort and why its denial still galls him. Compared to the value Vinnie placed in the public exoneration from blame symbolized by an annulment, the international legal fees were pocket change. While the Church's rebuff may once have forced Vinnie to take a long look in the mirror, whatever truth he saw there left no mark that I ever observed.

Vinnie next married Stella, also an Italian citizen. This marriage was doomed by Stella's father, an overbearing man whose murder Vinnie once plotted in some detail. After Stella lost a full-term baby, she suffered a mental breakdown and attempted to strangle her father when he arrived at her bedside. She had to be pried off his neck. Although Vinnie continued to remember her fondly 30 years later, he divorced Stella after she was institutionalized. Their son, Alberto, who bears the name of his paternal grandfather, was raised by Stella and her mother.

Vinnie again married an Italian woman three years after divorcing Stella, this time with the express goal of having children. The stormy marriage to Rita, who Vinnie compared more than once to the hurricane of the same name, lasted only a year and a half. Rita nevertheless served her "purpose" and bore Vinnie twin sons. One son was named for Vinnie's uncle, Angelo and the other was again named for his father Alberto. Barely four months later, the "neglectful and abusive" mother and wife abandoned her sons and husband and returned to Italy. Raising his sons became the focus of the next 20 years of Vinnie's life, an investment he felt yielded poor returns. "I had to sacrifice a great deal," Vinnie often repeated. "I've given up a lot in the world and have nothing for myself." Yet at Thanksgiving the year we talked, Vinnie's then 30-year-old sons and their partners arrived at his house bearing not only all of the food but entire toaster ovens and other equipment with which to cook it. The effort made to bring the festivities to the ancestral home was extraordinary, yet insufficient to satisfy Vinnie. Even days after she cooked his Thanksgiving dinner, recalling Angelo's wife's ultimatum that Vinnie would have to come to his son's house for the next family holiday prompted a tantrum.

In a world that Vinnie conceived of as friendless, his relationship with his twin sons represented the most important source of meaning. His mood fluctuated with the amount of attention Alberto and Angelo accorded him and the extent to which they bent to his will, performing the chores and tasks his illness prevented him from doing for himself. Vinnie therefore resented Angelo's wife and Alberto's fiancée. The women, for their part, sensed they were competing with the father for the sons' attention and were apparently eager to see Vinnie placed in a nursing home. In this battle, illness was one of Vinnie's main weapons, authorizing Vinnie's demands for his sons' attention in a way that the twins and their wives could neither challenge nor ignore. What they could do, however, was run from his demands. On the pretext of his wife's dislike for New England, Angelo moved to Florida midway through my time with Vinnie, an event he described as "a personal tragedy."

Another such tragedy was the loss of Vinnie's twenty year job as business manager for a ceramics manufacturer. Vinnie's ability to strike a bargain for the company was much appreciated by the owners. The arrival of a supervisor who resented Vinnie's authority and perks, however, marked the beginning of the end. Shortly after going over his boss' head to appeal for a raise and then showing him up by halving the cost of a six-figure contract for a new computer system, Vinnie was fired. At interviews for new but equivalent positions, he often broke down crying. During the succeeding years, Vinnie maintained his family in marginal circumstances, only rarely working at low-skill jobs or brokering the sale of an antique car.

The initial humiliation of losing his job compounded by the failure to bargain his way into a new one eventually demoralized Vinnie so badly that he virtually gave up on life, and he identified this as the starting point for his health's downward spiral. The death of his father soon after and, a few months later, a severe stroke suffered by his mother provided further trauma. Vinnie still wept when speaking of his parents and blamed this combination of stressors for an anxiety attack one Christmas Eve. The ensuing medical examination at the time identified for the first time his high blood pressure, low thyroid hormone level and diabetes. Diagnoses in hand, Vinnie confronted social adversity by becoming "sick." Adopting the "sick role," a status both invented and enabled by the medical system, allowed Vinnie to circumvent expectations that he overcome failed marriages, the loss of a job, and the death of his parents to provide for his children. Furthermore, illness represented an excuse for failure and a declaration of his helplessness in the face of more powerful forces.

Illness even provided Vinnie a forum to exhibit his talent at negotiation, scorned by his employer when they fired him and the potential employers who failed to hire him. He suffered a life-threatening episode of gastrointestinal bleeding when he developed an ulcer which bled profusely from the blood thinner he was taking to prevent clots in his leg veins. After weeks of feeling "spacy" and passing dark, tarry stools, during one of his multiple weekly visits for tests or appointments, Vinnie collapsed in the hospital lobby in shock from blood loss. After he recovered, the experience reinforced Vinnie's prodigious consumption of healthcare. "If I had been home and collapsed, I would have died. Being as I was coming to the hospital three, four times a week, saved my life," he told me. In other words, Vinnie believed that neither specific therapies nor quality care were keeping him alive. Instead, he correlated the volume of care he received with his prognosis. The goal of maximizing the amount of time he spent in the hospital involved convincing his doctors that he needed constant tests and referrals and gave him ample chances to employ the single skill of which he was most proud: negotiation.

Vinnie was an inveterate and skilled dealmaker. Getting more than his money's worth seemed to afford him real pleasure. The happiest I ever saw him was when he had a favorable bargain to report, as during our first meeting. Tired of his television, he had decided to buy a new flat screen model. Careful research in consumer magazines and on the Internet identified a mid-range LCD TV that got "three stars out of five" from one rating service. But unlike your typical shopper, Vinnie did not simply go to an electronics store to purchase the $1479 set. Neither did he search the Internet for the best deal or find a used model for sale. Instead, Vinnie gave a friend the money to buy a new one. On Vinnie's instructions, the friend returned the television to the store a day later claiming that it turned out to be too small for his wall. Sitting in his car in the parking lot, Vinnie waited until he saw store employees bringing the set back out to the floor. Striking up a conversation with the manager, he quickly established a rapport and began working his magic. The price for the "used" television eventually fell to $739. Vinnie recalled the precise before and after prices for his new toy with a tone of self-satisfaction and pride.

This pattern of behavior was not isolated to the television set, nor was the willingness inherent in it to cynically manipulate others for his own ends. During one clinical interaction, I listened to Vinnie wheedle his third round of free impotence treatments out of his urologist. Recalling a trip to the Dominican Republic to obtain a divorce, Vinnie proudly told of convincing the judge to shorten the process from the week that "celebrities and politicians have to wait" to just a few days. Among the other things that Vinnie acquired at below-market cost using persistence, patience, and blatant immorality were his living room furniture, a new patio for his house, and, not least, his medical care.

Vinnie received free medical care through the Massachu-setts "uncompensated care pool," a system since replaced by the state's universal insurance plan. In this program for people with income below 200 percent of the federal poverty line, hospitals and medical systems gave into a common fund that paid other hospitals to cover the cost of care not reimbursed by Medicaid or Medicare. At the time, the threshold for a single-person household to enroll in the pool was $19,600. Vinnie's annual income from renting out his house's enormous upstairs apartment—he charged perhaps two-thirds the market value—and Social Security totaled nearly $29,000. He had not paid taxes in four years. The ground-floor apartment where Vinnie lived was large, with beautiful wood flooring, high ceilings, and a refurbished kitchen. The furnishings were tasteful, recent, and expensive. The living room was outfitted with deep, com-fortable leather chairs and sofas, a massive television, and a professional-grade stereo system. A large cabinet held a gor-geous and valuable snuffbox collection. Two antique cars, in-cluding a black 1970 Corvette convertible in good condition, were parked in his driveway. Yet besides the free care pool, Vinnie partook of multiple other aid programs meant for in-dividuals and families living in poverty. He got assistance with his electric bill from the Salvation Army and heating assistance from his gas company. He did his grocery shopping by driving to multiple free food pantries, while complaining about the as-sortment of food offered. By obtaining free healthcare and, with the help of chronic illness, these other underserved ser-vices, Vinnie demonstrated to himself and other his value as a negotiator and as a person.

I observed how life events altered Vinnie's biological sta-tus, and his illness determined his life trajectory in ways that were far from purely physical. Life shifts were embodied as shifts in the course of his illness, whereas illness shifts were understood only on a background of life events. Vinnie reinterpreted both his illness and his life story constantly until the two were woven together into a single seamless fabric. The story of Vinnie's fourth marriage and the next phase of his health troubles was one of the largest designs embedded in this fabric. He began "researching" women of various Asian nationalities in an attempt to identify a companion for his old age. He decided to pursue Thai women who he felt, were attractive and obedient and could quickly learn accent-free English. At the age of 55, he became "pen pals" with a Thai woman named Vanida, who he said "was supposed to be the ultimate plan for my old age." To avoid "complications," Vinnie underwent a vasectomy before traveling to Thailand to wed his 22-year-old bride.

In order to sponsor Vanida's visa, federal rules required Vinnie to hold a job. He found a job driving elderly individuals to medical appointments. About a year after his marriage to Vanida, he developed chest pain after work. He did not immediately seek treatment, instead returning to work after a few days. Asking his son to wait around the corner with the car, Vinnie began preparing his van for the day but quickly returned to the office complaining of chest pain. He refused the staff's offer of an ambulance and instead called his son for a ride to Dr. Aronson's office, which ensured coverage by Workman's Compensation because the "onset" of chest pain occurred at work. He was initially sent home after a normal electrocardiogram but was called back when blood tests suggested a heart attack. Vinnie eventually underwent placement of a stent to open a blocked blood vessel.

Vinnie's convalescence proceeded slowly over the next year. Vanida proved to be an excellent caretaker but also took a job at a convenience store, something Vinnie had previously forbidden. Although she ostensibly sought employment in order to improve their financial standing, work outside the home allowed Vanida to escape the social isolation that marriage to Vinnie entailed. (When I once asked what he thought it was like for Vanida to marry a much older man and move to a foreign country, Vinnie could not even begin to formulate an answer.) Thai friends that Vanida met through work helped her win a better job at a local university. Given his vasectomy, Vanida's eventual pregnancy signaled his wife's infidelity to Vinnie in no uncertain terms. Finally, Vinnie traveled to a Caribbean island to obtain his fourth divorce. To say that the "stress" of this situation caused the Crohn's disease attack that sent Vinnie straight from the airport to the hospital is to say that the excruciating pain was a physical manifestation of severe emotional suffering. The Crohn's component of Vinnie's illness worsened to the point of hospitalization on both the first and second anniversaries of his final divorce.

Vinnie needed a dense social support network but operated in such a way as to ensure the consistent failure of his relationships. For instance, after they jointly inherited their parents' house, Vinnie condemned his sister for forcing him to buy her out rather than coming to live with him. He blamed her "devious" behavior on her exposure to "foreigners" who he said are getting free college degrees here. During another discussion, Vinnie told me he "wanted to make his sons understand that to get something they had to work for it." In both instances, Vinnie was able to offer up these opinions without apparent irony. For my part, though I struggled to receive these statements with a straight face, I knew Vinnie bore as little responsibility for his behavior as a patient with blocked coronary arteries bears for his chest pain.

Throughout my acquaintance with Vinnie, I tried to listen sympathetically as he revealed his intertwined medical and social struggles. But I often felt irritated or even angry with him, a failure reflected in the judgmental tone I saw and heard in my descriptions of this poor, sad man. At one point midway through our year together, I presented Vinnie's case for a class on how to take a patient history. As I spoke to this small group of classmates and faculty, all of whom I'd grown to trust, I astonished myself with my negativity. Why wouldn't he just get better? Why wouldn't he recognize the feelings of others? Why was he so *difficult*?

It is perhaps unsurprising that I should eventually come to think of Vinnie as difficult. "Doctors, find chronic illness messy and threatening," our professor Dr. Arthur Kleinman, the medical anthropologist, taught us. Predictably, the chronically ill become problem patients in care..." Physicians employ a variety of coping techniques with difficult patients, ranging from non-judgmental listening to referral elsewhere, from strict control of the doctor-patient interaction to withdrawal of their investment in the outcome. Doctors are not supposed to dislike their patients, and feel guilty when they do. This certainly describes the pattern of behavior I fell into: embarrassed and disappointed with myself for my aversion to Vinnie, I allowed myself to reduce the frequency of our interviews and to shift focus from continued interaction to writing and analysis. But rather than try to suppress the emotion, one of my advisors suggested reframing the issue in a new light: "These responses represent information as useful as the physical examination, because they provide important information about our patients or about ourselves." This evaluation required first bringing the emotions to awareness and subjecting the feeling to interpretation. Neither task is particularly comfortable. As I progressed through my medical training, I frequently thought of Vinnie. I realized that a physician who addressed only Vinnie's diseases—the elevated blood sugar, the inflamed bowel, the sclerotic arteries—would have failed to significantly improve his patient's health.

I once pointed out to Dr. Aronson that he saw Vinnie significantly more often than I saw some of my closest friends. He laughed and admitted that many years of clinic visits had helped him develop an empathic understanding of his patient that has proved important for his medical care. Dr. Aronson's success depended on maintaining a positive attitude about the potential for curative care while conceding that medical successes would likely not change Vinnie's manner of being in the world. I recognized all these things intellectually, yet in the years since Vinnie and I parted ways, I have found myself searching for better answers.

I have found myself drawn to a career in the intensive care unit, working with patients who are desperate to claw their way back to the kingdom of the well. It still feels wrong to reduce expectations, to accept that Vinnie's prospects were better in the kingdom of the sick. As I near the end of my training, my faith in medicine's flawed creeds is no longer blind, but has survived the test of Vinnie's heresy and others like him. I'm just not sure if this is a good thing or a bad thing.

Cheerful Bravado

JANINE KNUDSEN

Floyd is a seventy-year-old man with a lengthy history of strokes and heart attacks and a defibrillator implanted in his chest. He transferred to his current doctor, Dr. Mansfield, after transitioning out of the local Health Care for the Homeless program. As a medical student or resident on rotation in the hospital, this is the most I would probably learn about Floyd: a list of his medical problems and medications, and maybe a snippet of his social history. There is a chance that I might discover his passion for soccer, his deep eagerness to please his doctors, and his plans to donate his body to Harvard Medical School. But I would miss his generosity, his pride in his volunteer work, his ability to take both successes and failures in stride, and the many other qualities that make him who he is.

Floyd and I were introduced during one of his increasingly frequent doctor's visits. Before he arrived, I pored through his chart, attempting to soak in his long, scattered medical history. His many surgeries, medications, and medical problems blurred in my head, as I tried to link them back to the courses I had completed in medical school so far. As a picture of Floyd grew up in my mind, a man walked past me in the hall. He moved slowly, carefully, with a look of curiosity on his face. His tan, fall jacket hid a round body, and gave him away as a native New Englander. This then, was Floyd. When I followed Dr. Mansfield into his room a few minutes later, I was surprised to feel some trepidation. My familiarity with the elderly was mostly limited to my grandparents and close relatives. How was I expected to treat Floyd? How, in fact, do most doctors balance the deference and respect accorded to the elderly with the authority of their medical profession?

Dr. Mansfield answered these questions, and the many more that I was piling up, within minutes. She greeted Floyd with a balance of familiarity, concern, and professionalism that would have charmed even the most reticent patient, and deftly dove into an assessment of his medical concerns. Not that Floyd was an unreceptive patient—quite the opposite, I quickly learned! Polite, but visibly beaming, he exclaimed, "It's so good to see you!" Floyd's childlike exuberance at human friendships, and what I learned was a wonderful, and often overwhelming, eagerness to please, was not something I expected in the elderly. In fact, I soon found that the phrase "elderly," and all the associations I had with it, didn't fully seem to fit Floyd.

He clearly didn't think so either. "Old" was not a word in his vocabulary. As Dr. Mansfield conversed with him about his reasons for coming in, he described a variety of symptoms: worsening fatigue, shortness of breath, dizziness, and a fear of falling. Yet he never framed this in the context of aging, shying away from the label of frailty and decline. Was this naivety or a coping mechanism? Or was it, perhaps, perfectly normal?

The decline in Floyd's health is, like his life story, vague, gradual, and difficult to trace back. But certain milestones do stand out, both in Floyd's memory and his medical record. At fifty years of age, he experienced his first heart attack. Unfamiliar with and uninterested in the medical system, he took hours to seek medical care, and returned to work only days after his hospitalization. The next heart attack came when he was sixty. At work as a contractor in a remote location, he was airlifted to a hospital, where he spent four days recovering as an inpatient, only to fall through the cracks in the system again.

Soon after, Floyd became homeless, moved to Boston, and suffered two silent strokes. While this might seem like a trivial description for momentous life changes, it is the best that Floyd can offer. In 2001, he suffered a stroke that affected his frontal lobe; his personality and memory haven't been the same since. In the same year, a defibrillator was implanted in his chest, followed in later years by two cardiac stents to open up the blood vessels in his heart.

Coming up to the present day, Floyd is 70 or 72 years old, depending on whether you consult him or his medical chart. He is no longer homeless and lives in elderly housing, supported by Social Security and Medicare. His heart attacks have left him with congestive heart failure; in addition, he has developed peripheral vascular disease. Damage from his latest stroke, which temporarily robbed him of his ability to speak, gives him difficulty reading novels and recalling words.

While these brushes with death seemed like harrowing and life-altering experiences, Floyd describes them matter-of-factly. In my interviews and conversations with him, he delivered descriptions of his heart attacks, his divorce, and his experience with homelessness in a concise monotone. In contrast, his voice leapt with eagerness, betraying a small stutter, when he began to describe his vacations in Aruba, his volunteer work at a hospital Stroke Club, and, most touching of all, his choice to donate his body to Harvard Medical School.

In our first meeting, this dichotomy confused me to no end. Were the heart attacks not as bad as I thought? The strokes not as debilitating? Was congestive heart failure as mundane as high cholesterol? I couldn't see past Floyd's cheerful bravado. I listened, head nodding, as he spun off lighthearted stories about his love for soccer and his German heritage, and walked out of his exam room feeling as though I had gotten to know him well. A friendly, fairly healthy, elderly man, I thought.

In the following months, I began to see how inadequate my understanding was. As I followed him through his encounters with the medical system and built up my knowledge about heart and lung physiology, I came to realize the fragility of his condition and the amazing resilience of the human body and mind. With Dr. Mansfield's patient guidance and observations, I learned to notice problems Floyd left unspoken, to take note of nuances such as his gait and tone of voice, to read between the lines of his stories. In my courses, I learned about the underlying causes and lasting effects of heart attacks and strokes. All of this helped me develop a better grasp of Floyd's medical history, and a more sensitive eye for his fluctuating health.

Floyd was part of a culture I had all around me, but knew little about: the elderly. Unlike the field of infectious disease, where I spent most of my time before medical school, the goal of medicine is not to cure the patient and restore them back to their previous function. There is no "cure" for old age. Floyd's care was, therefore, about maintaining his quality of life as he aged, addressing his concerns and daily needs. End-of-life questions were much more salient as well, and I learned to become more comfortable with them. Those conversations came later, when I made a concerted effort to learn his perspective on difficult issues—from living with physical constraints to end-of-life decisions. When he introduces me to friends and acquaintances as his medical student, I always respond, lightheartedly but truthfully, that Floyd is my professor.

Heart disease is the leading cause of death in the United States, accounting for more than 700,000 deaths a year. Floyd was one of the lucky survivors of a highly prevalent and fatal condition. The estimated incidence of heart attacks in American adults is 1 in 150. Even more shocking is the mortality rate for each attack—a whopping 30 percent. Floyd, absorbed in his work as a contractor, uninformed about the warning signs or risks of heart attacks, and disconnected from the health care system, waited hours to seek care. When he finally did make his way to a hospital in Springfield, nurses measuring his blood pressure told him that it was sky high. He still nearly refused treatment. Perhaps he assumed that a heart attack should look and feel different. Hollywood and newspaper headlines tell us that heart attack patients seize up and keel over, that death is instantaneous. There is little information in the lay press about the slow progression of heart disease, as blocked heart vessels stop delivering blood to the hardworking heart and tissue begins to die. Nor is there adequate information about the confusing symptoms caused by our body's curious nerve structure, such as the radiating referred pain that Floyd felt down to his wrists. Thankfully, his doctors were able to convince him to remain in the hospital, where he ultimately stayed for three days.

During his hospital stay, Floyd became one of the success stories of great American medical care. A combination of medications and sound medical decision-making rescued him, making him one of the fortunate heart attack survivors. But on the other side of the coin, Floyd serves as a frighteningly common example of the considerable failure of our health care system. Longterm primary care was nonexistent for him, due to either the cost of insurance or the hassles, or both. Although million dollar studies such as the Framingham Heart Study have helped scientists determine risk factors for heart disease from smoking to high blood pressure to psychosocial stress—all of which Floyd had—there was no one to screen or counsel him. Not surprisingly, he became one of the millions of Americans who use the Emergency Department as their safety net care.

Over the next ten years, unbeknownst to him, Floyd's heart disease continued to worsen. Then, a few years later, he suffered from his second heart attack. If his memory serves him correctly, this was precipitated by a heated argument: In those days Floyd had a strong temper. At this point he had already divorced from his wife as well, and was living on his own, moving for each new commission.

Floyd's heart attack occurred while he was working on a bridge project in Massachusetts. One day, he remembers, he developed trouble breathing, especially when lying down. Again, he only sought care at a hospital after hours of discomfort. Although the medical details of this event are lost on him, he remembers being airlifted by helicopter to a hospital in New

Hampshire. This high-level intervention could only do so much, however; enough heart tissue had irreparably died during the period of ischemia that his heart function was seriously compromised.

Floyd currently lives with the diagnosis of heart failure. The ejection fraction of his left ventricle is less than half of what it should be. He also has peripheral neuropathy, or loss of sensation in his legs. Floyd, however, is his usual cheerful self. During our first few meetings, I had no understanding of the impact that heart failure was having on his life, in part because he was refusing to let it. Only in retrospect did I realize how much it could impede his daily activities, from walking to the grocery store to socializing with friends.

Scans of Floyd's brain, done a decade later, also show that he suffered two silent strokes around this time. These "silent" strokes, so named because they lack the classic symptoms of a stroke, are astoundingly common: among people with coronary artery disease such as Floyd, their prevalence reaches nearly 50 percent. Despite being asymptomatic, this tissue damage can cause decreases in cognitive and physical function.

While these sequelae often go unnoticed, they seem to have had serious repercussions in Floyd's case. Although the timeline is unclear, Floyd did lose his well-paying contractor job around the time of this event and was forced to move out of his home. The details of this transition are lost: Floyd can simply remember that he hopped on a bus to Boston and made his way to the Salvation Army shelter in Cambridge. He describes this experience in a matter-of-fact voice, not mentioning the word "homeless." Whether this represents his normalization of the experience, or perhaps his denial, is unclear; Floyd insists that he cannot remember any of it.

Whatever the reason, Floyd became a member of an extremely marginalized and underserved population. He was able to break the cycle of chronic homelessness, however, to access medical care and, eventually, find a home. Floyd finally received primary care for the first time in decades through the local Health Care for the Homeless Program (BHCHP). His physician at the program for the homeless, Dr. Holmes, left such a positive impression that Floyd expresses his gratitude effusively at every possible opportunity. Under Dr. Holmes' careful surveillance, Floyd received the screenings, checkups, and medications that had been unavailable for so long.

Floyd doesn't hesitate to mention that his doctor helped to save his life. While sitting with Dr. Holmes during what was now a routine visit, Floyd suffered a serious stroke. Exhibiting his usual tenacity and independence, he nearly refused Dr. Holmes' help, by attempting to walk to the emergency room down the street. Thankfully, Dr. Holmes convinced him to let the paramedics wheel him there—for with heart attacks, every second matters. Once there, Floyd was diagnosed with a severe stroke involving the frontal lobe of the brain. The frontal lobe controls such a wide variety of functions, especially those involving higher level reasoning, that it can be said to be the seat of our personalities, affecting motor function, problem solving, spontaneity, memory, language, initiation, judgment, impulse control, and social and sexual behavior. Without realizing it, I had observed nearly all of these in Floyd. From his difficulty recalling words in normal speech to his diminished control of impulses and thoughts, he experienced these aftereffects on a daily basis. His frequent complaint at Dr. Mansfield's office was his fear of falling due to his lack of balance, which made even short walks uncomfortable. Yet he had come a long way, achieving momentous improvements during a nine-month, post-stroke rehabilitation program.

One evening, I followed Floyd to his monthly "Stroke Club," of which he is a proud member. A wonderful concept, these meetings bring together stroke survivors each month for small charity projects. Some are more debilitated than others, but all share an excitement for seeing each other and contributing to the community. One month, they packaged Valentine's Day candy for the children's ward; another, they wrapped up scarves to give to breast cancer patients. Observing them for an evening, I realized how much worse Floyd's experience could have been. Many of his friends were in wheelchairs, struggling with movement and also speech. I also finally understood the strong sense of gratitude that he felt towards his doctors and rehabilitation specialists, who helped him so far.

At the end of our evening at the Stroke Club, he pulled me through the hospital's long corridors to meet his rehabilitation doctor. In Floyd's mind, this man seemed to stand out as a cross between a magician and a saint, and I had to meet him. Floyd had entered the rehabilitation hospital barely able to speak. It was as though he had a mouth full of marbles, he described, and the words just weren't there. Yet by the end of nine months, with his doctor's help, he had proved that his aphasia was surmountable. His memory still lags, but he explains that it was much worse.

This health was not to be taken for granted, I learned. Every visit with Dr. Mansfield was a balancing act. She tweaked his medications, monitored his defibrillator, listened to his heart, mapped his blood pressure; even the smallest changes required careful management, and there was little room for error. When I first met Floyd, this balancing act was slowly tipping in the wrong direction, with increasing consequences. His heart failure had started acting up, and he was putting on water weight. He could no longer work at his beloved volunteer post at the U.S.S. Constitution because of his worsening exhaustion, and was stuck at home watching soccer on television.

Soon Floyd's cardiologist decided that he needed to replace the batteries in his defibrillator, a device that was placed in his chest and delivers electrical pulses or shocks, if he has an abnormal heart rhythm; as a result of his damaged heart muscle, it was no longer working as it should. The battery change was an outpatient operation, brief and uncomplicated, and I was there to take Floyd home afterward. Although he had many acquaintances, he had no family to take care of him. His son, a 52-year-old real estate agent, had just moved with his wife to California, and his daughter no longer speaks with him. Although he is the eldest of seven siblings, only one lives in Boston. Floyd's support structure is now limited to a few acquaintances and his many doctors and nurses.

I found Floyd upbeat as always, sitting in the waiting room after surgery. He shrugged off my questions about pain and fatigue, and somehow convinced me to go with him on a visit to the U.S.S. Constitution. This ship, a relic of the Revolutionary War, was his pride and joy; he had been talking about it for months. In his time as a museum volunteer before his heart failure began to worsen, he showed it off to visitors from around the world, learning words in nearly twenty languages in the process. When we came by, it was a freezing winter day, but neither the weather nor his hours-old surgery dampened his excitement. He introduced me to all his old coworkers and dragged me through every inch of the museum. Oblivious to his need for rest, I followed him everywhere, excited to see him in his element.

A few days later, I accompanied him to his cardiologist for a follow-up appointment. When I met him at the bus stop, he was nearly unrecognizable. Unshaven, with rumpled clothes and dusky skin, he explained that he had been unable to sleep for the past three days, because getting in and out of bed was difficult. I assumed that he hadn't had much chance to eat either. An enormous blue bruise had also spread around the site of his surgery, although his doctor described this as normal. I was shocked to realize how greatly I had underestimated the fragility of the elderly, and how naïve I had been to let Floyd pretend that, at 72 years old, he could walk out of an operating room and on to a tour of the city. I was also reminded of the effects of Floyd's social isolation. With no family to care for him, he had practically been stranded at home, unable to perform simple tasks.

He improved over the following weeks, but his fragility stuck in my mind even more than before. At our next meeting, I finally confronted him with the difficult questions I had been too shy to ask previously. I wanted to hear his perspective on end-of-life issues and on living with chronic illness, themes I had discussed intensely in medical school classrooms, but never with real patients. Somewhat worried about how he would react to such sensitive topics, I felt a huge relief when he seemed unfazed by my questions. He had not, I learned, signed an advance directive or a "do not resuscitate" form, but could see their value. He also wasn't afraid of dying, despite his many brushes with death. After all, as he reminded me, he has already signed away his body for donation to Harvard Medical School. Only a few months out of the incredible experience of anatomy class, I was fascinated and moved by the sense of fulfillment that this decision gave him.

One day in March, weeks later, I learned from Dr. Mansfield that Floyd had been admitted to the hospital. He had arrived at a checkup visit with dangerously low blood pressure and she sent him to the hospital. This lack of blood pressure was making it harder than ever for his heart to pump out the correct volume; he needed fluids and medications immediately. Dr. Mansfield wanted him there for a night of surveillance, until she could arrange for a cardiac outreach worker to check in on him regularly. The city of Boston, I was learning, had a number of valuable resources for its elderly. Floyd was already receiving free housekeeping services from the Boston elderly association, and his quality of life greatly improved as a result.

I set out to the hospital the next day and found him sitting calmly in his room, his eyes directed at a soccer game on the television screen in front of him. I had spent the day worried about what this hospitalization meant for his declining health, and felt a rush of relief at not finding him bedridden and debilitated. He almost looked his usual self, although slightly the worse for wear. But when he jumped out of his seat to tell me he was feeling fine, I finally knew better than to take him at his word.

He explained exactly what had happened: He had taken a leftover pill that he found at home, which his pharmacist had noticed, and that he had alerted Dr. Mansfield, who called him in for an appointment; also, per usual, he had refused to go to the hospital, but Dr. Mansfield had finally persuaded him. Once in the emergency room, Floyd recounted, he was hooked up to so many tubes that he couldn't get out of bed. "I was there from two to nine!" he exclaimed, "without a bite to eat!" A few hours and a turkey sandwich later, he was doing much better, energetic enough to joke around and make friends with his nurses. As usual, it was human company, more than anything else, that helped him get back to his usual self.

When I visited him the next day, he was preparing for another heart study before his discharge. Dr. Mansfield had also come by to see him and was working with the emergency room doctor to change his prescriptions. "All the medications I've been taking, they're finally showing their wear," Floyd explained to me. "They also gave me four IV drips!" Calmly he added, "My kidneys are failing on me too, I guess."

He continued to tell me about how excited he was to get home after his night in the hospital. His neighbor, an elderly man in much worse condition, had kept him up all night, crying. "I heard them telling the family that he's dying, so I shouldn't give him a hard time," he admitted. After reflecting for a second, he added, unexpectedly, "I don't feel that way. After this, I'm going to Harvard!"

"Does that make you feel better?" I asked.

"Yes, it does. Really, it does."

Taking Things as They Come

CARLA HEYLER

When I was a freshman in high school, my grandfather was diagnosed with multiple myeloma, which is a blood cancer formed by the overgrowth of malignant plasma cells that crowd out the normal blood-forming cells. Very few treatment options were available to him and he passed away several years later. While my grandfather's illness was the initiating factor that led me to pursue a career in medicine, I had never taken the opportunity to learn about course of his disease. When I received the opportunity to work with Anne, a patient with multiple myeloma, I was unsure of how this experience would affect me.

During the course of my visits with Anne, it became apparent that she did not understand her illness or her treatment. At one point I asked her to explain multiple myeloma to me, and she admitted that she did not know anything about what cancer was or how it began. She attributed this to her coping mechanism of "taking things as they come," and explained that she knew equally little twenty years ago when she was being treated for breast cancer.

At one visit, we started talking about the treatment she was undergoing, the many treatments she had already undergone, and about the future. She confessed how tired she was from so many different protocols and how intense it was to take part in a clinical trial. She worried that this treatment would not work. When I asked her what it meant for a treatment to work, she explained that she hoped to go into remission.

Later, I met with Dr. Ramsey, my mentor and the clinical researcher overseeing Anne's trials. Realizing I had never been told Anne's prognosis, I asked Dr. Ramsey to explain it to me. That was the first time I understood that Anne was going to die. Dr. Ramsey took out a graph labeled "The Natural Progression of Multiple Myeloma" and pointed to "refractory illness." There were no more plateaus; refractory illness was the last climb. Anne, he explained, would have to continue active therapy for the remainder of her life. With therapy, Anne would have at most 1 to 3 years to live and at least 6 to 9 months. Without therapy, Anne would likely live for only a few weeks. The goal of treatment would be to keep her numbers stable while maintaining her quality of life. Once the numbers began to rise, they would know that current therapy was no longer working and would commence with a new treatment. In other words, Anne's cancer was at a stage that, by definition, meant she would not go into true remission. She would always be maintained on treatment that was not intended to cure her but, rather, was experimental in nature.

I was suddenly struck by the fact that Anne had switched from her local physician to a physician that was over an hour's drive away, in order to enroll in this experimental treatment that involved more frequent visits and more research-driven procedures, rather than patient care. She was enrolled in studies designed to test the maximum dosage of new therapies, and had been experiencing side-effects so severe that she was unable to leave her house. In response, she chose to reduce her dosage, but was afraid that reducing it too much would eliminate its effectiveness. And above all, she either did not or chose not to understand the fact that she would have to continue receiving new treatments for the rest of her life. Afraid I would overstep boundaries I imagined between Dr. Ramsey, Anne, and myself, I did not bring up these issues. I was at a complete loss for what to do and felt caught in a moral dilemma.

Sometime later, I had the opportunity to watch "Wit" (a movie based on the play by Margaret Edson), which became a turning point in my understanding of Anne's situation. Wit follows Vivian through her eight-month battle with metastatic ovarian cancer, or, more accurately, through her eight-month battle with treatment for metastatic ovarian cancer. Wit addresses several ethical issues surrounding clinical research, particularly those that arise for terminally-ill patients whose only treatment options are clinical trials. This is known as "therapeutic misconception," when research subjects assume that a therapeutic intent exists in clinical trials when, in fact, it may be that such trials will not benefit them at all.

A clinical researcher and a doctor wear different hats: A doctor wears the cap of beneficence, intending to provide therapeutic treatment in the present; a clinical researcher wears the cap of beneficence for the future, intending to provide therapeutic treatment at some later point in time. That is not to say that clinical researchers intend to harm; in fact, they are bound by ethics not to. But there is a very real conflict that researchers experience when on a quest to expand scientific knowledge. After all, doctors treat patients while clinical researchers study participants; the inherent therapeutic nature of a patient-doctor relationship is removed in a clinical research setting. While clinical researchers hope that a therapy will be therapeutic for participants, their intention is to demonstrate with certainty whether a therapy will be therapeutic for future patients. Here is the conflict: On the one hand, clinical researchers do not intend to harm, but on the other, they are motivated to encourage individuals to enroll in trials, to push through negative side effects, to take unbearable doses for the sake of scientific conquest. And that is exactly what happens in Wit: Whether intentionally or not, Vivian's physician presents the trial as "the best treatment we have to offer you," as if it is intended to treat her stage-IV metastatic cancer. And, as if it is a bonus prize, he adds that she will be contributing to scientific knowledge. As Vivian has just been told she has terminal cancer, what is she supposed to do? She is vulnerable. She cannot possibly know that, in the end, she will die of her treatment, not her cancer. Furthermore, the doctor tells her that she must withstand the full dose of therapy; in his words, "There may be times when you wish for a smaller dose, but we have to go forward with full force." At what point does the harm become greater than the benefit? And along those lines, to whose benefit are we referring, the patient's or the researcher's?

I cannot say that I know the exact answers to these questions, but they gave me food for thought and some insight into Anne's position. I still believe that clinical trials are necessary for medical progress. They have produced treatments that have allowed Anne to have a longer and better quality of life than ever could have been expected 50, 20, even 10 years ago. Anne has said that being enrolled in a clinical trial makes her feel as though she is able to give back, to contribute valuable information that may help others. The care that Anne has received has been paid for by study sponsors, and included beneficial procedures that might otherwise have been deemed unnecessary. Her care has been delivered with impeccable attention to detail, and has, in her own words, been "extraordinary, professional, and personal." Moreover, the staff is comprised of deeply caring, committed, intelligent, perceptive individuals who possess an optimism that is refreshing in a field that could otherwise so easily become oppressive. In fact, Anne modeled her pseudonym for this casebook after individuals who have been involved in her care, all of whom she looks to for guidance when making decisions about her care. So it is definitely not that clinical trials are bad, and it is certainly not that the people who design clinical trials are bad; in this case, it is, in fact, quite the opposite.

After watching Wit, I realized that the issue I was struggling with was a challenge that clinical researchers and patients alike face. It was not a personal thing that could be attributed to Dr. Ramsey, and it was in no way indicative of him as a human being; it was simply the nature of the proverbial beast. And so I decided to talk to him about it. I was a bit hesitant and introduced the topic with a question: "Do you think it would be a good idea to focus on some of the ethical considerations of clinical trials for my paper?" To which Dr. Ramsey responded with, "Absolutely. The main ethical consideration is the use of clinical trials as treatment, and what factors go in to making the decision to participate." He continued by emphasizing that, at the end of the day, the patient comes first: "It's the coldness of the intellectual process that we need to be very careful to avoid, and, at the end of the end of the day, the guiding principle should be what is best for the patient." From his point of view, being a clinician and being a researcher are not incompatible; clinical trials either should be seen as therapeutic or should not be conducted in the first place. We also discussed patient comprehension and coping mechanisms. He emphasized the importance of recognizing that patients have many different ways of facing their illness and of cultivating trust within this context. At the end of the day, one must respect and maintain the very delicate balance between helping patients to understand and letting them approach understanding in their own way. This conversation did not clear up all of my concerns regarding clinical trials, but it certainly made me feel more grounded in relation to Anne. While Dr. Ramsey's position may seem optimistic, he truly embraces the role of both clinician and researcher, expressing genuine excitement not just for the outcomes of a trial but for what those outcomes have meant, in terms of each individual patient.

Throughout the course of this year, I realized that becoming a doctor is inherently about making diagnoses, about learning to transform a chief complaint into a treatment plan, with the ultimate goal of achieving "good health." In the process of making a diagnosis, you meet a person. And it is, I believe, the meeting of that person that defines the difference between being a diagnostician and being a physician. The beauty of medicine is that a day in a white coat means a day spent meeting people, people from whom you can learn not just by listening to their stories, but by listening to how their stories are told. Anne taught me as much in what she said as in what she did not, shared with me a picture made of pieces that she let me put together again. In taking a step back from this puzzle, I could see that medicine is ultimately learned from the patients; the classroom is merely supplemental to this process.

Medical school is not just a time for growth but for learning how to grow, and that the white coat is not just a thing to be worn but must be earned. Doctors are human, medicine can be uncertain, and finding an answer is not always the answer. From Anne I have learned about trust, not just how to give it, but also how to receive it. I have learned about vulnerability. I have learned that uncomfortable can be a good thing, that complicated does not even begin to explain it, and that silence can sometimes be the best interruption. But, above all, I have learned that every patient will be a new person to meet, a new story to be told, a new lesson to be discovered.

And that is a beautiful thing.

ACCEPTANCE

We must be willing to let go of the life we have planned, so as to have the life that is waiting for us.

— E. M. Forster

Beyond Alphabet Soup

PRIYANKA SAHA

She looked up at me with those wise dark brown, eyes, staring steadily into mine. They seemed to be infinitely deep, imbued with a maturity and wisdom far beyond her young age. They were eyes that had already experienced more pain, shed more tears, and developed more endurance and grit than adults many decades her senior. Yet her eyes showed calmness and serenity, a knowingly controlled resignation to the reality of the pain she would have to suffer to repair the broken body she was given at birth. These were eyes that disarmed, but also mesmerized, many an adult with their sage and steady gaze.

On first glance, the precocious wisdom of her eyes was the only thing that betrayed the fact that Jessie was not your typical year-and-half-old baby. Jessie was a normally growing baby, meeting all her normal milestones, and had even outgrown the need for early intervention at home. She was steadily building her vocabulary, starting with simple words, like "Mommy," and slowly inserting them into sentences. She was energetic and playful, allowing a bit of mischief to glimmer in those brown eyes from time to time and always smiling, ready to make a new friend.

The reason behind her premature share of pain and those precocious eyes was a congenital disorder called VACTERL association. The term VACTERL is shorthand for structures and organs that the disorder affects: the spine, rectum, heart, breathing and swallowing tubes, kidney, and arms and legs (Vertebral, Anal, Cardiac, Tracheo-esophageal, Renal, and Limb). Patients with this condition are each unique, and their symptoms can range from nonexistent or minimal to severe in each letter category. Most children with VACTERL undergo numerous corrective surgeries. However, VACTERL association does not cause any mental problems and is not progressive, and thus the overall prognosis is quite good.

For Jessie, her condition involved all the letters of the disorder except for "TE"—tracheo-esophageal—defects (breathing and swallowing). She was born with heart defects that required immediate surgery after birth. In total, her heart required three surgeries for a full repair. Her spine and limbs were only moderately affected. She showed outstanding motor development in standing, sitting, and walking. If highly observant, one might notice the right thumb wobbling freely at its joining with the hand, devoid of fine motor control. The thumb was completely dislocated from her hand, and prevented her from having the function of an opposable right thumb. She had only one functional kidney and urinary incontinence, which would require corrective surgery later in life.

Perhaps the most devastating anomaly for Jessie was her rectal defect. She was born without the muscular control of the anal sphincter to hold and release stool, and had fecal incontinence—leaking stool without control. Her anal opening was also abnormally small. For this reason, Lydia had to manually dilate the opening of Jessie's rectum on a daily basis, which caused both her and Jessie significant pain and discomfort.

VACTERL is more than just an assortment of letters and list of anomalies. Beyond experiencing every physiological consequence of the disease, Jessie endured the daily pain of rectal dilatations, countless pokes and prods of examining doctors and nurses, and the sting of healing wounds induced by the surgeon's scalpel. Jessie's mother, Lydia, also shared equally in the emotional distress that the disorder causes. As Jessie's devoted and doting caregiver, Lydia felt every stab of pain as acutely as Jessie did. Because of her young age, Jesse could not communicate with me in words about her experiences, so Lydia became her voice and my primary source of their experiences. Mother and child became one as the patient.

The journey they took me on was truly one of unforgettable lessons that I could not have found anywhere else in my first year of medical education. Together they showed me what it means to suffer an illness, what it means to be a mother and advocate for one's own, how tragedy can strain relationships but also build strength, how crucial and fragile lines of communication across the healthcare team can be, and how the latter affect the patient-doctor relationship.

I was told that Lydia was a "difficult mother"—that she yelled and screamed at nurses when her baby was sick; that she had tried to fire doctors when things weren't going right. I took this information in with some trepidation. I was worried that it might be hard to talk to Mom and develop rapport. Perhaps she would yell at me too and shut me out. But I reminded myself that she agreed to have me follow her baby's care and share experiences with me, and that it was a privilege for them to let me enter their life.

I decided I was ready to take on the challenge of getting to know my patient's supposedly disagreeable mother. After all, this is one of the challenges of Pediatrics, people had told me. Treating young kids invariably comes with communicating with parents and families, in times of joy as well as in times of frustration. At the time, I could only vaguely imagine how tough it must be for parents to see their children suffer from illness and how their fear and worry might transition to frustration and anger under certain circumstances in the doctor's office.

Needless to say, I was honestly a bit nervous before my first encounter with my patient, Jessie, and her mom, Lydia. I sat in the waiting area of General Surgery, staring expectantly at the doors through which Jessie and Lydia would enter. I knew it was them when they came in. Mom, a tall and broad-shouldered woman in her mid-to-late 30s, came in pushing a black stroller. I smiled up at her and she smiled back; she knew that I would be coming to the appointment. She parked the stroller next to a chair and lifted Jessie into her arms.

My heart warmed immediately at the sight of Jessie, with her sweet, dimpled smile, tuft of curly brown hair, and her calm and innocent brown eyes, recently awakened from a nap. With a small sigh, Jessie rested her head against her mother's chest and calmly looked at me with a purely serene and content expression on her face. Lydia looked completely at ease with her baby in her arms, and happily chatted with me while we waited to be called for the appointment.

In that moment, any and all nervousness that I had harbored before melted away. Gone from my mind were the images of a combative mother. In fact, I could not imagine a happier, more agreeable mother and child coming in for a pre-op visit. The scene of baby Jessie resting in Mom's arms was to be a frequent sight in my future encounters with my patient and her mom. Seeing Jessie in Lydia's arms reminded me of a painting from Hindu tradition, of baby Krishna resting in the arms of his mother, Yashoda, similar to renditions of the Virgin Mary caressing baby Jesus—images epitomizing the highest and purest bonds of motherhood. From that first moment with them, I was convinced of the complete devotion and dedication with which Lydia loved Jessie. I would see countless examples of her love and the strength of her motherhood. I would come to learn that Lydia was not a "difficult" mother; she was a tenacious mother, a mother with an undying love for her baby, a mother who would do anything for the wellbeing of her child.

It was during that first preoperative clinic visit that I caught a glimpse of the pain that can accompany motherhood. Because Jessie's rectum was not connected to her anal sphincter normally, she was unable to control bowel movements, and also did not have the muscle tone in her rectum to maintain an appropriate opening of her anus. In order to maintain the size of her anus for stools to pass, Lydia was required to use dilators—plastic rods with increasing diameter— to manually dilate Jessie's anus at least once a day. As uncomfortable as one can imagine it would be for Jessie to receive the dilatation, I soon realized that it was equally, if not more, painful for Lydia to perform the dilatations. It was a daily ritual for them that involved Jessie thrashing her tiny limbs and tears flowing from both mother and child.

In the surgeon's office, Jessie was smiling and happy, until her mom went to remove her diaper. It was clear that she knew what was to come. She had been conditioned into fearing diaper changes, because they were sure to involve the painful dilatation procedure. She shrieked and kicked out her legs as Mom placed her on her back and cooed gently into her ear. The surgeon also tried calming Jessie, as Mom prepped the first dilator and brought it towards Jessie's anus, holding it like a pencil.

I caught myself holding my breath as I watched Lydia, and tried to process what she must endure every day to ensure that her baby could poop—something that most of us take for granted! She went about it with a resigned look of determination on her face, and I marveled at Lydia's fortitude. As soon as it was over, Jessie was reaching for Mom again, and Mom was quick to take her into her arms. In talking with Lydia later on, I learned how frustrating it was for her to have to dilate Jessie's anus daily. It hurt her to see her daughter in distress, even more so because she knew that she was the one inflicting the pain.

Motherhood comes with immense responsibility, and as I learned that day, that responsibility sometimes carries with it immense pain. I was reminded of examples from my own childhood. Growing up in the protective cocoon of my mother's love, it was often my mom who was the first to let out a gasp of pain if I had fallen down. Her eyes would be fighting back tears as I hollered at the sting of alcohol on a scraped knee. She would be by my side with a Band-Aid at the slightest hint of a paper cut. I often still tease my mom about these incidents, and joke laughingly that it was as if she was hurt, not me. Yet, now I wonder if it is in fact true. Perhaps mothers do feel real pain when their child is hurt. I could certainly believe it after watching Lydia and Jessie.

Jessie was diagnosed during an ultrasound when Lydia was six months pregnant. The news was devastating. "Why me?" Lydia wondered constantly. She could not justify why someone like her, a hard-working woman who makes healthy choices—she does not drink or smoke—should have a complicated pregnancy. In the initial days after the ultrasound, feelings of sadness and anger bubbled inside of her. Lydia underwent many different tests, including an amniocentesis and stress test. She "drove herself crazy" by reading about the condition on the Internet, although doctors had warned her not to.

At one point, the doctors asked her whether she wanted to terminate the pregnancy, because she only had two weeks before it would no longer be safe to do so. She fleetingly considered it, wondering whether she was mentally, physically, and financially prepared to care for her unborn child. However, these hesitations passed quickly because she could not imagine not bringing her child into the world. She fiercely embraced her pregnancy and did not look back. She took care of herself, ate well, and was very healthy. She gained 15 pounds and felt amazing. She never had any swelling or morning sickness, as she had with her previous three pregnancies. In fact, Lydia was working nearly up until the day of her delivery.

The delivery, however, was not without complications. She was admitted for an emergency cesarean section. Lydia's last recollection before the cesarean procedure was that Jessie's heart had stopped beating, and she thought that her baby had died. When she awoke from the surgery, she found, to her relief, that Jessie was alive but would need heart surgery immediately. Anxious to be with her newborn baby, Lydia rushed in to see Jessie after the first operation. It was a full open-heart surgery, and upon reaching Jessie in the intensive care unit, Lydia nearly passed out. She was overwhelmed by the sight of Jessie's tiny body connected to so many tubes and machines. She had not expected to see her in such a state.

Jessie spent the following two months—the first two months of her life—in an induced coma to keep her quiet and safe while her heart healed. This was perhaps the worst two months of Lydia's life. She was severely depressed and physically ill. Lydia describes herself during that time as a "complete mess." She was sick with vomiting, diarrhea, and was unbelievably stressed and anxious. Following Jessie's birth, Lydia could not eat and she vomited up anything she consumed, including water. She lost a significant amount of weight, lost a lot of hair, and the cesarean section incision did not heal properly. She constantly feared for Jessie's life, and began to fear that she would be burying her little baby in her grave and planning for her funeral. Her doctors stressed to her that she had to take care of herself, because she would not be able to care for Jessie otherwise.

Slowly but surely, with the help of family and doctors, Lydia continued to get better and stronger each day. What Lydia says ultimately helped her escape the dark period of her life was her own conscious choice to heal and to be strong. When I asked how she did it, Lydia laughed and said, "I don't know." Her father tells her that she's a superhuman, and she seemed to agree—with a bit of humble disbelief– that she is a superhuman mom. She has her stressful days when she feels frustrated and overwhelmed, days when she wakes up and cries and finds it hard to get up and get going. But then she prays and resolves that it's what she has to do, and so she will do it, and that she is not alone. Lydia is utterly devoted to Jessie, and says that she will do whatever she has the capacity to do for her daughter for the rest of her life. Jessie gave her a new purpose in life and made her, and continues to make her, a better person.

Lydia's situation made me recall how I wept uncontrollably at the end of "A Temporary Matter," one of the short stories in the award-winning *Interpreter of Maladies* by Jhumpa Lahiri. The story, which I first read during high school, is about Shukumar and Shoba, a Bengali couple living in Boston, who silently drifted apart after the death of their first baby. One week, a series of scheduled power outages in their neighborhood forces them to be in each other's company during dinner every night. In the darkness, they begin to reveal small confessions to each other, and gradually they regain the intimacy they had lost. With each power outage comes greater intimacy, and the reader (in this case, me) becomes increasingly hopeful that their marriage might be saved.

On the very last page, when Shoba reveals her final confession, that she had decided to move out, the hope for them that I had created came crashing down around me. Quite unexpectedly, tears emerged fat and heavy from my eyes and rolled down my face in steady streams, as I wept with Shoba and Shukumar "for the things they now knew." I was bewildered by the suddenness of my reaction, but more than that, I remained utterly confused as to why the marriage, whose rescue seemed so promising, had abruptly come to an end. Why had the death of their baby catalyzed such a downward spiral in Shoba and Shukumar's relationship? Why hadn't their shared grief brought them closer together? Surely, if I were in Shoba's place, I would have reached out to Shukumar and sought each other's comfort, right? In my teenage naiveté, the reasons behind marital distress were completely beyond my understanding.

One of my conversations with Lydia caused me to revisit some of those questions and to think about how marriage is affected when tragedy strikes, especially tragedy concerning a child. The first time I spoke with Lydia, I noticed that she rarely mentioned a father-figure in Jessie's life. Tentatively, I had asked her about Jessie's father, feeling slightly uncomfortable and anxious about potentially opening up old wounds. She briefly told me that she was still married to Jessie's father but that they no longer lived together. Things had gotten too heated and hectic around the time of Jessie's birth and first surgery, and so they decided to take a break. I was surprised and saddened to hear of the separation and wanted to ask her more questions: I wanted to know if the father still came to see Jessie, whether he showed that he cared for her, whether they were on speaking terms. I wanted to know how Lydia had managed to become a single mother, caring for three more kids in addition to Jessie, during such a stressful time. But, at the time, I felt uncomfortable to probe further and so I let my questions subside.

On a later date, I told Dr. Meili what I had learned about Jessie's family situation. Dr. Meili was not as surprised as I had been to hear that the tumult around the time of Jessie's birth had led to separation between Lydia and her husband. She claimed that this was, unfortunately, a common occurrence in families when they discover the diagnosis of a serious illness in their child. I found this observation to be curious and sad. It was still perplexing how the strings of a strong marriage could unravel so quickly and so suddenly.

In March, I attended a conference for families and caregivers of children with complex health needs. At least a few hundred people were in attendance at the large event, occupying several floors of Boston's world trade center. It did not take long for me to notice that the overwhelming majority of attendees were women. For the most part, these were mothers of children with various medical complications. At one of the conference workshops presented by a mother of a daughter with a rare genetic disease, I again noticed, as I had while talking to Lydia, that there was very little mention of any father-figure. Like Lydia, this mother spoke proudly of a strong network of extended family but hardly said a single word about a spouse or partner.

At the final workshop of the day, I began to get some answers. The workshop was on transition planning for families of children with special healthcare needs—on how to address questions of independence, guardianship, further education, and more for their children. One of the workshop leaders was herself a mother of a child with a complex health condition. From the time of her son's birth to about age seven, her life was a constant race to and from the hospital, in and out of surgeries and doctors' visits. Like Lydia, she also had several other children to look after; but unlike Lydia, she had her husband by her side throughout. It was not until her son was about seven years old, when his medical problems seemed to calm down somewhat, that she realized there was something wrong in her marriage. She found that she could no longer sit down and have a normal conversation with her husband, eat regular meals with him, and be alone with him without having something medically complex to talk about. They began seeing a marriage counselor to try to sort out the barriers that had come up between them.

It was in marriage counseling that she learned something so profound, yet so obvious, that it almost amazed her that she had not realized it herself: "We were no longer a married couple. Instead, we had become a crisis management team," she said, "and our job was to put out fires. When there were no more fires to put out, we didn't know what to do with ourselves." Thinking about what she had said, I realized that, when faced unexpectedly with a seemingly insurmountable challenge, couples have a choice to make—they can either choose to confront the challenge together as a "crisis management team" or they can choose to cope individually. The choice seems simple enough, perhaps even obvious, that the practical choice would be to fight together, to gather strength through company, but in reality it is not so easy. Challenges, like the birth of a medically complex child or a death of a family member, can bring to light certain differences or incompatibilities that make the jump in roles from married couple to crisis team a challenge in its own right. For Lydia and her husband, the incompatibilities had been too great for them to put out the fires together. Her husband was not good at handling difficult situations, she told me; Jessie's birth overwhelmed him.

Once things started to return to some normalcy, Jessie's dad started to be more present in her life. While clicking through photos of Jessie and her other children on her phone one day, Lydia came upon a photo of a giddy Jessie playing with her dad. Sandra, Jessie's nurse-practitioner, mentioned that Jessie sometimes came to appointments with her dad instead of her mom. Lydia mentioned that he even came to the house everyday to help out. It made me happy to hear that her husband was trying to incorporate some of the responsibilities of crisis manager while returning to his role as husband.

I am usually not one to reread books or stories multiple times, but for some reason, "A Temporary Matter" captured a part of me that led me to revisit the story on more than one occasion. Perhaps because the characters were from the same ethnic background as me, I felt an immediate kinship with Shoba and Shukumar, both first-generation Bengalis growing up in America. Perhaps it was the similarity I saw between them and my own parents, who had also suffered the pain of losing a child in infancy, and of having another—my older sister—with a complex healthcare need. Perhaps it was my conviction that all marriages have the potential to be resilient and fixable, especially one like Shoba and Shukumar's, which seemed to be so close to resolution. In any case, I picked up the story once more, and thought again about what I had learned from Lydia.

It was as if I was reading the story for the first time. It was suddenly perfectly clear to me why Shoba and Shukumar were destined for separation, why their incompatibility was so impossible to mitigate, why they could not be a crisis-management team. In grieving their child's death, Shoba and Shukumar realized they both wanted two very different things: The stillbirth left Shoba yearning more than ever for the chance to be a mother, but it left Shukumar with the cold realization that he was not yet ready to be a father. The opposing desires had driven a stake through their marriage. The signs were there all along, and I finally had the eyes to see them in the story and accept the truth for what it was without judgment.

It was finally the date of Jessie's long-awaited study to see if her bladder and urethra were functioning properly, so that Dr. Meili could appropriately plan the rectal surgery. I arrived a bit early to the clinic, eager to observe my first full procedural encounter between Jessie and her caregivers. Having a few extra minutes, I looked around the waiting room and realized I was the only one there. The room was small but equipped with several chairs, both large and small, to accommodate its guests. The smaller chairs surrounded play tables, some containing built-in Etch-a-Sketch boards or magnetic games. Against one wall was a small bookshelf stocked with both new and well-loved picture books waiting to be picked up. On the wall next to the bookshelf was a "Creative Kids" art gallery showing off the talents of the many kids who had come to the clinic. The room was filled with the sounds of PBS programming coming from the television hanging from the ceiling next to the reception desk.

I was quietly absorbed in the TV program when Lydia and Jessie entered. Jessie was calmly bundled up in winter gear and appeared to have just awoken from slumber. Lydia undid her winter coat and hat to reveal a shirt proudly stating, "Grandpa's Girl." "That's her favorite man!" Lydia happily chuckled.

122

Jessie was quickly drawn in by the picture books and waddled over to the bookshelf. I noticed that her gait had gotten steadier and agile since the first time I saw her in October. I joined her at the table with some picture books, and happily passed the time until a nurse called her name. The nurse led us into a narrow corridor towards a scale to get Jessie's height and weight. Jessie happily obliged as she tottered onto the scale. The nurse read off her height and weight—Jessie was showing excellent growth!

From the height and weight station, we went into the examination room for the study. The room was dark except for a few fluorescent lights around the room, the glow of the computer monitors, and one large central lamp over the examination table. I was struck by how large the examination table was. As they placed Jessie onto the table, it seemed as though the table would swallow her up. I wondered why they had such a large table for a baby so small. Wasn't it a *children's* hospital? And what a contrast from the vibrant and cheerful waiting room! There, the colors were brighter and the tables smaller, to match the children for whom they were designed.

There were three women in the room. From what I could tell, they were nurses. They had Lydia undress Jessie from the waist down to do a perineal exam. They told Lydia that they would be inserting a catheter into Jessie's urethra, to determine whether the urine was coming directly from the bladder, and an electrode to determine nerve function. As soon as the women began examining Jessie's perineum, the crying began, and would continue in heart-wrenching bouts punctuated by resilient spells of silence for the next hellish hour. The women tried repeatedly, without success, to insert catheters into Jessie's tiny urethra. They tried to distract her by playing a video of "Dora the Explorer" on the TV monitor, which was conveniently placed above the exam table looking down onto Jessie's face. Lydia waved a light-up princess wand near Jessie's face.

But Jessie would not quiet down. The bubbly, happy, and easy-going baby, who so willingly played with me in the waiting room and obliged the nurse at the weighing station, could not be comforted. I could not help but imagine how painful the procedure was.

The scene was, in a word, nightmarish. My body was tensed and my senses were on overload. In front of me I saw three grown women in blue surgical gowns trying with all their might to contain the tiny, squirming arms and legs of a 16-month-old baby. As I stood near the foot of the table, I saw the bright light of the lamp bring Jessie's perineum into harsh focus. I saw the blood-red swabs of antiseptic used to paint the vaginal area strewn on the table after being used. With each swab, my ears registered a shriller shriek from Jessie's overworked vocal cords. The sight, combined with the painful wails of the baby girl, was violent. The only sounds adding some minimal element of relief or calm to the situation were the constant vocal reassurances from the nurses and Lydia. She quietly stood at the head of the table, her torso bent over her daughter's head, her face next to Jessie's tear-streaked one, one hand stroking her hair, the other offering fingers for her to clasp.

It was one of the most difficult encounters I have ever witnessed, and somehow the nature of the procedure and the delicacy of the area of the body that was being studied made it even harder for me to witness. I marveled at Lydia's calm composure as I watched her huddled over Jessie, offering her the comfort of her touch. She had told me before how hard it was to see her baby suffer, and for the first time I was experiencing the pain she had described. I moved around the table to stand next to Jessie, and placed my hand next to Jessie's free hand to hold onto. The tenacity with which she grabbed my hand expressed to me how much discomfort she was in.

Sometimes I find it hard to reconcile the different personas of children's hospitals: Waiting rooms in bright primary colors and decorated with images of friendly animals; musical notes emerging from the walls with every step up the stairs; and lobbies outfitted in the newest of technological gadgets to capture the attention of young and old— children's hospitals take on the guise of a playground, nothing less than a corner of Disneyland carried back to major cities such as Boston. But beyond these colorful waiting rooms and lobbies, behind the singing walls, are anxious parents awaiting a doctor's diagnosis, crying babies, and nervous children uncertain of what their future may hold. Unlike Disneyland, the hospital is not a place children beg their parents to take them to. Why, then, this act of treachery, a magician's illusory trick, disguising a hospital as a playground?

I was abruptly reminded of this harsh reality as Jessie's pained wails filled my ears. What had seemed to start out as a daydream filled with sounds of "Dora the Explorer," sights of sparkling lights from a toy princess wand, and the comforts of picture books had quickly turned into a nightmare. Finally, at the end of the dark hour, and after a quick debrief with the doctor, Jessie was free to go. When Jessie reemerged from the dark confines of the urodynamics study room, I was surprised to see how quickly she regained her cheerful, content 16-month-old demeanor. It seemed that she had already swept aside the unbearably painful hour she had endured moments before, as she quickly padded over to the small bookshelf strewn with picture books once more. Her grandmother—who had just joined us, Lydia and me—looked on with smiles at her innocence. I wondered if children have blissfully short memories of pain. Or, perhaps, was this her way of expressing her victory? She had emerged from the doctor's arena a champion, having conquered the many challenges set for her. The colorful waiting room laden with books was her prize, welcoming her with open arms and cheers of applause.

What had been a cacophonous hour ended on a sonorous cadence. Baby girl was happy once more, and Mom and Grandma (and I) breathed a sigh of relief. In this cadence, I gained a new appreciation for the dress-up game that masks the somber and often painful dealings that go on behind closed doors. The colors and sounds are more than just a disguise. They are a message of welcome, a cheer of motivation, and resoundingly hearty congratulations to the brave and valiant fighters who enter and exit the hospital every day. They are pillars of moral support, a means of saying, "We care and we're there for you." Toys and games may not lessen the pain and suffering induced by procedures, and may not alter the reality of illness, but at least they can be a symbol of care and love.

Last spring, Jessie and Lydia struggled with a rash that had developed on Jessie's bottom. Due to Jessie's frequent swings between diarrhea and constipation, the skin around Jessie's vaginal and rectal area became irritated and inflamed. There were open sores and cuts all over her bottom. Dr. Meili, her surgeon, had seen her about the "diaper rash" in January and prescribed a few ointments and creams. The rash responded well to the topical creams, particularly one that provided a thick moisture barrier. However, Lydia soon ran out of the appropriate cream, and the time period that followed was one filled with frustration and miscommunication, as Lydia tried to acquire more. The saga of the cream and diaper rash is a complicated one, and one that I gathered from multiple points of view, each with its own highlights and perceptions.

When the cream first ran out, Lydia called Jessie's pediatrician to inquire about getting more. Unable, for whatever reason, to provide this cream, they gave her a series of other ointments to treat the rash. They tried treatments for fungus, yeast, and bacterial infections, but the rash did not resolve. Lydia kept asking for the original cream, knowing in her heart that that was the only thing that would work for Jessie. Dr.

Meili was not informed of the rash or that Lydia was unable to acquire more of the effective moisture barrier cream.

Without the proper cream, the rash on Jessie's bottom got worse and worse, to the point where the open sores prevented Jessie from being able to sit up. Lydia recalls that Jessie would cry constantly, not being able to eat or sit or play or excrete wastes without pain. With each passing day without the proper treatment, Jessie became more fitful and Lydia more anxious and frustrated.

In retrospect, Lydia wished that she had thought to contact Dr. Meili's office directly for more cream, instead of going through the pediatrician's office. After all, Dr. Meili was the first person to have examined the rash and prescribe the cream. Lydia felt that the pediatrician had not assessed the rash properly and, thus, had not provided the right kind of care. Had Lydia contacted Dr. Meili directly, perhaps she would have been able to obtain the cream much sooner, and Jessie's rash would not have been as severe. Unfortunately, the news of the severity of the rash did not reach Dr. Meili's ears. Instead, between May and June the problem only worsened and made Jessie sicker. She had multiple emergency room (ER) visits due to diarrhea and vomiting, which may or may not have been related to the rash and the discomfort it caused.

Jessie was finally admitted to the ER due to fever and a urinary tract infection. The pain with urination was so significant that Jessie had stopped urinating regularly, which Lydia thinks contributed to the infection. This was ER visit number five, and "finally they started taking me seriously," Lydia told me. Lydia had kept trying to tell them at the ER that the only treatment that ever seemed to work for the rash was the moisture barrier cream, which was only given to Jessie at the hospital, and she could not obtain at home. At the hospital, Jessie's rash was treated with oatmeal and Demboral soaks and the proper cream and the rash immediately began to resolve.

Two weeks later, however, the rash started to come back—with a vengeance. At this point, Lydia was overcome with panic. At the time of discharge, Lydia was not given any of the cream to take home. She was told that Jessie could only get it while being treated at the hospital. Lydia did not know what she could do to prevent the rash from recurring again and a-gain, without resorting to admissions at the hospital for access to the proper cream. In a frenzy, Lydia began making phone calls to any and all of Jessie's doctors. Lydia called her ped-iatrician's office to try to get in touch with Dr. Meili's office but could not get an immediate appointment. She then asked to get some cream from the office in the meantime, but says that she was denied a prescription because the "medication is only pro-vided in the hospital." Lydia then tried calling Urology but was unable to reach anyone. She finally reached one of the nurse practitioners in the clinic at the hospital, Sandra, who under-stood the severity of the situation and wrote a prescription for the cream, so that Lydia could get her own supply for home. She also bridged the communication gap with Dr. Meili. As soon as the doctor learned about the difficulty in getting the cream, she made sure to help Lydia get an abundant supply.

Lydia remembers being a "hysterical mom" during this dark time period, especially when the rash returned two weeks after the hospital admission, She cried in the hospital, yelled at doctors and nurses, and "felt like no one was helping" and that "no one understands how I feel as a mom." She was frustrated and upset because her baby was in so much pain. According to Lydia, the prolonged period of misery and frustration over the lack of the proper cream was largely a consequence of miscommunication within Jessie's healthcare team and could have been prevented. She did not want to blame any one doc-tor because proper communication is a team sport and re-quires everyone's efforts. However, she felt that information about Jessie's rash was not relayed to the right ears and that no one had listened to her properly. Lydia also admitted responsibility for some of the miscommunication, acknowledging that she should have called Dr. Meili's office directly rather than calling the pediatrician in the beginning.

There may be more than a little truth to Lydia's comments about information transmission across Jessie's team. "She tried to fire me," Dr. Meili told me with a chuckle, as she recounted her side of the story. By this point in the timeline, Lydia was at her wit's end and frantically called Dr. Meili's assistant demanding to see a new doctor. Dr. Meili was utterly bewildered by Lydia's frantic expressions over the phone, and felt extremely sorry for all that they had had to go through. From Dr. Meili's end of the story, once she found out about the rash, she took measures to connect with the nurse practitioner in primary care and make sure that Lydia could get the cream. Lydia later apologized for her outward frustration that she let out on the hospital staff members. Dr. Meili also apologized for the miscommunication and for the delay in resolution.

Although the lapses in communication had some role in the mishandling of the cream supply, there was more to the story than perhaps Lydia or Dr. Meili knew. I learned a third angle to the story from Sandra, the nurse practitioner in the primary care clinic. Sandra's role is invaluable to moms like Lydia. She is a direct liaison to other doctors and source of information and comfort to parents when they contact the primary care practice. For Lydia and Jessie, Sandra provides the "glue" that connects all the pieces and players of Jessie's care at the hospital together. When I asked Sandra about the diaper rash story, she explained that a large part of the confusion stemmed from communication issues with the cream's distributor and with billing. Although Sandra had a written letter from Jessie's insurance company stating that the cream was approved, the company representative verbally informed Sandra that the cream was not approved, and thus did not pay the pharmacy. Because the pharmacy could not distribute the cream before receiving payment, delivery had been greatly delayed. As it turned out, apparently the makers of the cream also had other inherent issues with their delivery system. Nearly a year after the diaper rash saga, Lydia still continued to face significant problems receiving shipments of the cream to her home. Fortunately, she worked out a solution of stocking up on cream through Dr. Meili's office to avoid a sequel to the infamous incidents of the previous year.

The story of the skin cream highlighted a more systemic issue about communication. Throughout my first year of medical school, there was one piece of advice that nearly every patient I encountered shared unanimously: *listen* to your patients, they told us, because your patients know and understand their bodies better than anyone else. Being Jessie's mother, Lydia has a finely tuned intuition about Jessie that, it seems to me, is often underappreciated by providers at the hospital. Lydia knew from the start that more of the proper cream was the solution to the problem, but instead was taken on a roundabout path of antifungal creams and ED visits and unanswered phone calls. Perhaps if she had spoken from the start with Sandra, the nurse practitioner, or Dr. Meili, people Lydia claims really heard and understood her, she would have found a quicker resolution.

Still, there was something more troubling to me about this story. Why is it that, time and time again, the one thing that patients find most distressing is being unheard by their providers? Why is it that countless well-intentioned physicians, nurses, and care providers are committing the same mistake of not listening? Surely, if so many are falling victim to the same problem, there must be something more systemic at play. No one enters the field of medicine or healthcare with the intention of not listening to patients. In fact, the most common corollary to the ubiquitous theme of "I want to help people" of medical school application personal statements is "I like to listen to people's stories." If these are the sentiments that draw people to medicine, then where do they go in practice when a patient is present in the flesh? Am I also doomed for a similar fate of receiving patients' worries with deaf ears?

I do not have answers to all of these questions, but I do have my theories. Perhaps some of the inattention to patients comes from the very training intended for treating patients. Perhaps in the years of focusing on numbers and figures and long Latin names and differential diagnoses and treatment protocols, empathy and listening are crowded out. Perhaps the newly acquired knowledge and the glimmering letters appended to a newly minted doctor's name imbue the sense that, because s/he knows more than the patient, s/he also knows better than the patient. My hunch is that none of this happens intentionally or consciously to belittle the patient, but perhaps is a pernicious side effect of medical education. It comes out subconsciously in little, seemingly benign ways: "Let's try another cream that's similar. It should work just fine," instead of "I hear you; that particular skin cream worked the best for the rash. We are trying to obtain it as soon as possible. How about we try an alternative to try to make things better in the meanwhile?"

What makes a doctor great is not how much they know or how many plaques they have hanging on their walls. The truest and highest honor any doctor can receive is the seal of approval from their patients. Sometimes being able to make a patient feel heard is the best and only thing a doctor can do. It is important for this message to be conveyed to medical students throughout their training, and even beyond medical school, so that they too do not fall victim to desensitization.

I feel fortunate to have had a first-year medical school experience that regularly reminded me to listen attentively. Whether by quoting the words of Francis Weld Peabody or by demonstrating exemplary patient-doctor interactions in clinic, our teachers made it clear the heights of excellence we should strive for. Unfortunately, listening skills are not always enough to provide the best care. Outstanding care also requires smooth coordination and hand-offs between caregivers, a perfect game of catch where the ball never hits the ground.

Jessie's surgery to repair her tethered spinal cord was also not a perfect game of catch. Lydia and Jessie showed up bright and early, at 5 a.m., on the morning of the originally scheduled date, expecting to be the first family in for surgery. Minutes and then hours went by, and they continued to wait. Jessie had been fasting since midnight and continued to not eat in anticipation of the surgery. Around 8 a.m., Lydia demanded to know what the delay was all about. It turned out that the original OR reservation had been made for a room that did not have the proper equipment for a heart patient like Jessie. The surgeon's office duly rescheduled the surgery but unfortunately forgot to notify the family of the change in date, which led to the logistical mishap.

Understandably, Lydia was very emotionally distraught by the situation. She told me that she cried and was depressed for the following few days. I imagined how frustrating it must be for a mother—who is already anxious about putting her baby into surgery—to be denied an expectation of care. The surgeon was also upset by the mishap made by his scheduling office, and made a great effort to get Jessie into surgery as soon as possible. Within two days of the original date, Jessie was in for the tethered cord release, and this time everything moved like clockwork.

This story highlighted the importance of meticulous coordination across providers, and how lapses can have amplified effects on the family. A rescheduled surgery might be as simple as rearranging a few names on a spreadsheet for a surgeon's office, but for the family it might mean asking the boss for a day off work, losing a whole day's worth of salary, calling a baby-sitter to watch the other kids at home, and spending sleepless nights in anticipation of seeing one's child being wheeled into the operating room under the veil of anesthesia.

I also came to understand how animosity is engendered between patients and the health care system. Miscommunication, mistakes, and mismatched expectations lay the seeds for distrust and dissatisfaction, even when, as often is the case, providers have the best intentions at heart. According to Lydia, her relationship with Dr. Meili had initially gotten off to a rocky start. First there was the chaos of the skin cream. Then there was a period of relative inactivity in which Lydia felt that Jessie's doctors were ignoring her needs. Lydia's one goal with Dr. Meili was to repair Jessie's rectum so that she could have normal bowel movements. Lydia's expectation was that the surgery would be scheduled without delay. She did not expect the surgery to be postponed further and further, pushing it into the following year.

The initial reason for delay was that Dr. Meili wanted Jessie to have a full neurological workup with the spine surgeon, to get a clear understanding of the anatomy of her nervous system before operating. The workup confirmed that Jessie's spinal cord was tethered and would need a repair operation. The second reason for the delay was that there was significant debate between Dr. Meili and the spine surgeon about whether the tethered cord release should be done before the perineal operation. Dr. Meili was of the mind that the spine surgery should definitely be done first, whereas the neurosurgeon did not think it was necessary. The delay caused by the back and forth between Dr. Meili and the neurosurgeon was compounded by the fact that it was summertime, and both Dr. Meili and the neurosurgeon went on vacations, one after the other. While the doctors were having discussions behind the scenes, Lydia faced silence on her end. She read the situation as one of being ignored by the medical team and of needs and expectations not being met. She felt some bitterness towards Dr. Meili for being unavailable, even though, unbeknownst to her, Dr. Meili was trying to be as thorough as possible with Jessie's pre-operative care to minimize complications.

During one of my first conversations with Lydia, she expressed her gratitude for the neurosurgeon for finally taking action and going ahead with scheduling the spine surgery. She was not as effusive then in her appreciation for Dr. Meili. The misunderstandings from the summer colored her level of satisfaction with her care, even though they had barely met more than a few times. Knowing how Lydia initially felt towards Dr. Meili, it was a really heartwarming experience to see how much her attitude towards her changed by the end of the year. Lydia ultimately developed a much more open rapport with Dr. Meili and now has the utmost gratitude for Dr. Meili's warm and friendly personality and detailed, yet easy, way of explaining things to her. She told me that it definitely makes a difference that Dr. Meili is also a mom, and that she understands at least some of what it means to be the patient's mom in such a situation. She could not express in words her gratitude for Dr. Meili and how glad she was that Jessie was being cared for under her guidance.

Being with Lydia through this transformation of her relationship with Dr. Meili made me realize how important the maintenance of relationships is to the care of the patient. Sometimes the attitude of the physician is all that a patient or family member sees, and may make the difference in whether the patient chooses to stay with the doctor. It also made me acutely aware of the many factors that influence patient's perception of a doctor, some of which may not be entirely within one's control.

A few months after surgery, Jessie was hospitalized for eight days for an infection of unknown cause. She came in to the primary care clinic on the morning of her scheduled rectal dilatation procedure for a quick checkup. Lydia had noticed that Jessie's fingers had felt colder than usual and that her lips had been slightly blue for a few days. In the primary care office, the nurses were alarmed to find that Jessie was running a fever of 104 degrees. Lydia was equally shocked and wondered to me later how she had not felt the fever when she touched Jessie. In addition to having a fever, Jessie's oxygen levels were low. She was immediately admitted for fear that her heart repair might be failing and that she would need additional heart surgery.

After a thorough examination of her heart, the team was relieved to confirm that Jessie's heart looked completely fine. They were not sure, however, about what was causing the fever. Lydia suggested multiple times to the doctors and nurses that it might be a urinary infection, since Jessie was prone to getting those and since the incision near her urethral opening was still healing. Lydia explained to me in exasperated tones that the medical team had repeatedly insisted that they place a catheter, but that she had to explain over and over that Jessie's bladder was too small for catheterization. She lamented the fact that people at the hospital were always so hesitant to listen to her ideas, even though she was usually right. After several tests, it was confirmed that Jessie, indeed, had a urinary infection, as Lydia had suspected from the start. I was reminded again of something we had learned in Patient-Doctor I class, of the importance to always elicit the patient's "explanatory model of disease," because patients often understand their bodies much better than we think. I internalized the lesson again, hoping that someday I would not fall into the group of skeptical medical professionals reluctant to hear a mother's theories for her sick child.

Over the course of her stay in the hospital, Jessie was given antibiotics and oxygen. Lydia complained that the hospital staff did not seem to have any plan, and that the doctors barely came by because Jessie seemed to be doing fine. She felt that they would keep her in the hospital until her oxygen levels improved and Lydia worried that they would be there indefinitely. I hoped that that would not be the case but, rather, that Jessie was being kept until the antibiotic course finished. Indeed, Jessie was allowed to go home the day after her antibiotics were completed.

I met with Jessie and Lydia on the seventh day of their stay. Lydia had remained at Jessie's side for nearly the entirety of the past week, going home only to shower and change clothes. She expressed to me that she was feeling "antsy" and "batty," due to being confined by the small hospital room. She had not been able to go to work all week, could not bring her own food to eat because of specific rules of confinement, could not take care of her other kids, and had very little company. Taking time off from work is expensive, not to mention arranging for childcare for the other kids; and I imagined how a weeklong stay at the hospital could cause financial strain, even while having adequate insurance for medical care. I understood why Lydia was concerned that the weeklong stay might transform into something much longer, if the doctors waited for Jessie's oxygen levels to increase. Lydia had oxygen at home that she had been trained to administer, and was confident that she could manage Jessie's care at home.

As I sat there in Jessie's hospital room, I noticed how freely Lydia conversed with me. Each time we met, she would greet me with a hug and smile. She told me I could ask her anything I wanted. I came out of each interaction with rich stories of their experiences and a sense of kinship and closeness. However, in between our meetings, there had been irregular pauses in our communication that could stretch for days or even weeks, periods during which I felt like the closeness had dissolved.

Unlike the experiences that some of my classmates were having, in which they met their patient nearly every week, my meetings with Jessie and Lydia were more sporadic. I mainly saw them at appointments with Dr. Meili, which were few in number and scattered across the calendar, or at other special appointments, such as the studies of her bladder function, termed urodynamics. Between these studies in December and the imperforate anus repair in February, we had absolutely no contact. I had tried calling multiple times but with no response. Soon I became absorbed by the rigors of medical school and did not make as strong an effort to get in touch. The same thing happened after Jessie's imperforate anus repair until her first postoperative visit several weeks later.

I felt guilty about it. I know that I personally struggle with maintaining contact with friends who live far away, and whom I have not seen for long stretches of time. "Out of sight, out of mind," my mom would quip, to alert me to my fault. Had I done the same with Jessie? Is this the kind of doctor I would be? One who would not remember her patients when they were not in front of her eyes? I knew it was something I had to work on, so I tried to come up with workable solutions. I wrote notes for myself on post-its and on my calendar, to remind myself to contact Lydia. Text messages being easier to deliver than phone calls, I began sending Lydia texts instead of calling her. I found that Lydia was also better about responding to texts than to phone calls. These were not perfect solutions, however. During one of the intervals between meetings, I stopped getting responses from my repeated text messages. I later found out that Lydia's phone was broken; Jessie had a little bit too much fun playing with it, and she had not had a chance to fix it.

When Lydia did not respond to my text messages on the morning of a scheduled dilation, I thought perhaps she was having phone difficulties again. I waited a week before texting her again, completely oblivious to the fact that she had been in the hospital for the past week with Jessie. I was shocked when my simple text of "How's Jessie? How are you?" was returned with the response "Things didn't go as planned on Friday and we have been admitted in the hospital since then. . . . Jessie got very sick." My heart skipped a beat as a hundred questions went through my mind: Is Jessie okay? What happened? What does "very sick" mean? Why hadn't anyone told me? The last question was especially stinging. I felt guilty once more for not being at their side when they most needed support. I also felt frustrated and slightly indignant that Lydia had not thought to text me when things had gone unexpectedly the previous Friday. I thought that we had developed a connection that would allow her to feel that she could contact me whenever she wanted. I thought she would want to keep me in the loop. When I got to the hospital, I reassured Lydia that she should not hesitate to reach out to me and that I would be happy to hear from her. She thanked me, and I hoped that maybe it would make a difference, although I doubt it really did.

The remainder of the year passed without any remarkable events and, also, with minimal contact. I tried to ask Lydia multiple times about setting up a meeting at home to see Jessie in her element, but somehow she always avoided answering. I sensed that she was not comfortable with having me at her house so I let my request drop. The barrier that I had sensed early on never quite went away. I realized that there could be many reasons for it. For one, I realized that Lydia was surrounded by an extensive network of extended family and friends to go to for support, and that perhaps I was just merely another well-wisher. I could understand that it might even be bothersome to her to have to remember to notify me, an outsider, of every change in Jessie's health. I also realized that her slight aloofness might have to do with how she viewed my role. As a medical student, I was neither a typical hospital visitor nor a doctor. While I tried to be her friend and shadow, I was also her doctor's mentee. Perhaps it was the wariness that I might have dual interests that caused Lydia to keep her guard up.

I may never know the true cause behind the hiccups in our communication throughout the year, but at least I can try to be content with some likely ideas. I also realized that developing openness with a patient is much more difficult than I thought. While some of the guilt that I felt is justified, due to my lapses in making attempts at communication, open communication must always be mutual. Only then can the loop be closed.

I woke up with a thrill on the morning of Jessie's surgery. It was finally the day that Jessie would have her rectum repaired. At long last, Jessie would have an anatomically normal bottom, and soon enough she would be able to poop at will, without the need to be dilated painfully every day. I ate quickly and rushed over to the hospital to meet with Lydia and Jessie in the pre-op area. Jessie was sitting peacefully against a stack of pillows on a large hospital bed with Lydia, Grandma, and Auntie by her side. Multiple doctors and their fellows came and went with consent forms to be signed. They greeted Lydia and smiled at Jessie, and matter-of-factly stated all the risks and benefits of the procedures that they would be doing. In- between signatures, Lydia, Grandma, and Auntie took turns taking photos of Jessie reclining like a diva on the bed. I offered to take a few photos of them with Jessie. Lydia explained that she wanted to create a photo book documenting Jessie's incredible journey.

Suddenly, tears began to fall silently from Lydia's eyes. They were tears of joy mixed with some tears of trepidation, I knew. The previous day, during Jessie's bowel prep—to clear all the contents of her GI tract before surgery—I had asked Lydia how she was feeling about the surgery. She had answered positively that she was quite excited. She had waited for this moment for a very long time and was excited and relieved to get it over with. Nonetheless, sending one's child into surgery under the spell of anesthesia is certainly never accomplished without some anxiety, and I was sure that there was some nervousness behind Lydia's tears as well.

Dr. Meili arrived around 7:30 a.m., delayed significantly by the snow-induced traffic of one of Boston's worst winters in history. We went up to her office to quickly review the procedures for the day and to collect scrubs. As I donned my scrubs, I thought back to my first experience in shadowing during an operation. It was the first operation of the day, and I nearly fainted. With a deep breath, I told myself that that would not be the case today, because I had eaten a hearty breakfast, and by now had seen several surgeries without feeling the slightest bit woozy. In the OR, we were joined by a party of others. There were nurses, technicians, and three other surgeons. One of them was Dr. Meili's fellow. Another was the urologist who would be doing the urological repair. The third was his fellow.

When we arrived, Jessie was already under the anesthesia, laying flat on her back on the surgical table. She was intubated and I saw her small chest rise and fall steadily. The room was equipped with two large monitors that would display a close-up video of the surgery in real time. Two more monitors displayed Jessie's vital signs in large bright colors and squiggly lines. As the team busily prepared for surgery, I tried my best to blend into the surroundings and not get in anyone's way. "Don't touch anything blue!" one person warned me good-naturedly, alerting me to the sterile field designated by the blue drapes around the instruments and on Jessie's body.

Finally, the surgery began at 8 a.m. and went continuously until 3:30 p.m. The urology team went first, using a sophisticated scope to inspect Jessie's anatomy. After a thorough examination, the urological surgeon and fellow proceeded to correct the abnormalities and create one vaginal opening.

An anesthesiology fellow sitting at the head of the surgical table explained the stages of Jessie's cardiac repairs in great detail. It was the first time that I had heard a thorough explanation of what exactly was wrong with her heart. I was riveted by the short cardiology lesson, soaking in as much information as I could, like a thirsty sponge. I also became the unofficially anointed photographer of the day. I eagerly obliged, humbled and slightly nervous about the opportunity to "assist" in the procedure. By the time the urology team had finished, three to four hours had already passed. Dr. Meili offered me a quick lunch or snack break, which I happily accepted. I was amazed by how she maintained her stamina throughout the procedure. Besides the small cup of yogurt I had seen her eat at seven-thirty in the morning, she did not have any other food or take any breaks until the operation ended at 3:30 p.m. I asked her later if she ever got hungry or tired during surgery, to which she responded that surgeons tend to live in a different state of time during surgery. Time speeds up and you don't ever feel the pangs of hunger or thirst that you normally would otherwise. I listened to her in awe, doubting whether the frequent eater that I was would ever be cut out to be a surgeon.

The anal repair was beginning just as I rushed back to the OR after lunch. I watched as Dr. Meili guided her fellow through the surgery, speaking to him as her colleague rather than her junior. She was an incredible teacher. She was neither overbearing nor aloof as she supported him throughout the delicate procedure. They meticulously divided the vagina from the rectum and created a new anus. It truly was a transformation. By the end of the procedure, Jessie gained the semblance of a normal bottom. It was beautiful. And I smiled as I thought of how happy her mother would be.

As the anesthesia team prepared to wheel Jessie to the intensive care unit, Dr. Meili and I left the OR to find Lydia. I learned that she and the other family members had been regularly notified of progress updates throughout the operation. Dr.

Meili greeted them with a huge smile and congratulatory note that the operation had gone really well. Lydia was elated and clearly relieved. We went into a small meeting room to discuss next steps. I watched as Dr. Meili skillfully explained to Lydia what the operation had accomplished. Lydia was the perfect student, following every word. She had several questions, which Dr. Meili answered with expertise in plain English, so that everyone in the room would understand. It was an incredible experience to watch the exchange especially knowing how Lydia had initially felt about Dr. Meili. As we said our goodbyes, Lydia gave us both huge hugs and expressed her joy and gratitude.

We walked back to Dr. Meili's office, a happy bounce in my gait from the emotional high of having witnessed such a momentous and successful surgery. As I would find out in subsequent visits with Lydia and Jessie, it truly was a significant milestone in Jessie's life. After the surgery, Lydia continued to dilate Jessie's anus regularly for a few weeks in order to maintain its patency and prevent it from closing. However, after a post-op visit with Dr. Meili, they decided to put a stop to the dilatations. Dr. Meili decided that in place of doing daily dilatations, she would look at Jessie under anesthesia in the OR once more in a few weeks and dilate her under anesthesia, to prevent her from feeling the pain and discomfort. What a relief! Finally the torment that had plagued Lydia everyday for nearly a year-and-a- half was coming to a close. Since the surgical repair, both Lydia and Jessie have been doing well. They are both free of the torment of regular anal dilations. As long as Jessie passes stools the "consistency of toothpaste," Lydia and Dr. Meili will be happy. Jessie can now tell her mom when she needs to go "poo-poo," so that her mom can sit her on the toilet. Despite the control over voluntary stools, she will continue to require regular doses of laxatives to keep her at a happy medium between constipation and diarrhea.

As for her heart, Jessie looks completely fine at the moment. Mom is planning for an early autumn date for the next heart surgery, so that she can heal before winter, since Jessie is especially prone to upper-respiratory infections in the cold. Jessie should eventually have a near-normal functioning heart. I wondered whether she might ever need a heart transplant, to which Jessie's cardiologist answered that, perhaps, in thirty to forty years, *maybe* she will need a transplant, but nothing can be said for sure.

Although the urinary incontinence and dislocated thumb are not so worrisome to Lydia at the moment, she knows that Jessie will need further surgery to fix those problems. The list of surgeries that Jessie has gone through and still must go through seems endless, but Lydia knows there is light at the end of the tunnel. She envisions a normal childhood for Jessie, for her to go to school and make friends and to run and play like normal kids. She also knows that Jessie may never be able to have children of her own, a difficult conversation that she must have with her at a future date. Lydia initially felt stressed at the prospect of having to explain VACTERL to Jessie and what it means for her future, but she knows it will be fine when the time comes. The hospital staff has been supportive and taught her how to have such conversations. Nonetheless, Lydia sometimes wishes that she was part of a larger network of parents who had had similar experiences with VACTERL.

I wondered how I would say goodbye. Saying goodbye had never been easy for me. I met with Lydia and Jessie one last time. I would miss those wise brown eyes and her dimpled smile. Lydia asked if it was permissible to stay in touch even after the year ended. I was delighted to hear her ask that! I had also wished to tell her that I would love to stay in touch if she was willing. I gave Lydia a big hug before turning to catch a ride back to the medical school. I felt happy and relieved. This was not a goodbye after all. This was an opportunity to further build a relationship—to continue to be a well-wisher cheering Jessie along on her journey and learning from her and Lydia.

A Favorite Chair

AAKASH KAUSHIK SHAH

As I rode the skip-stop elevator up, I was unsure of what to expect. I had spoken to Mr. Jones over the phone just briefly. His primary care physician, Dr. Rale, had called him to confirm that he was willing to have a first-year medical student, me, touch base with him from time to time so that I could learn more about the patient experience. Upon confirming, Dr. Rale allowed me to introduce myself to Mr. Jones over the phone. His voice was filled with a warm and welcoming mix of curiosity and enthusiasm. He immediately tried to get a sense of me as a person, in much the same way a physician with great bedside manner might. He asked me where I was from and what I did in the years before I came to Boston. Not wanting to take up too much of his time—I had gathered that dinner was already on the table—I answered, with a few quick sentences, and expressed my gratitude for his willingness to work with me. He then preempted my suggestion that we meet in person, by extending an invitation to his apartment overlooking the Charles River.

And so there I found myself, just a week later, taking the elevator up to his apartment, knowing little more about Mr. Jones than the fact that he was in his late 70s, lived with his wife, and had been diagnosed with diabetes a few years back. I had deliberately postponed looking at his medical file until after my first visit with him, so that it wouldn't color my perceptions of his story. Since I was enrolled in a course on how to interview patients at the time, I reasoned that meeting him before reviewing his file would also provide a good test—or, more accurately, practice—of my ability to take a thorough medical history.

His wife answered the door and led me into the living room, where Mr. Jones sat in his favorite chair. Ms. Jones went into the kitchen to prepare some tea and an array of sand-wiches for the three of us, while I took a seat in the chair just off to the side of Mr. Jones. As I looked around the room, I no-ticed that it was filled with keepsakes from their younger years, an eclectic collection of objects tied together by a life-time of memories and sentimental value. Photos, especially those of family, covered the walls and packed many of the shelves in the apartment. Mr. Jones was a natural storyteller. Each time he caught my eyes gazing at one of the photos, he would let out a knowing sigh and then launch into the tale behind it.

A photo from a family reunion taken under a bright blue, cloud-free Northern Minnesota sky took him back to his child-hood. I soon learned that he was born in a small town of 10,000 in 1931. He went to a Catholic school until the eighth grade, after which he entered the local public school. We joked about the kind of unsuspecting moments, often seemingly trivial ones, that leave a lasting imprint in our memory banks. For instance, out of all the important and formative times in his high school years, the one thing he remembered most clearly was his crush on Sheila Smith in the ninth grade. Upon spotting me steal a glance at memorabilia from his alma mater, the Mas-sachusetts Institute of Technology, he started telling me about how he enjoyed his years there but felt academically adrift. He was in the math department and joked about how his profess-sors taught him how to swim, since their teaching methods amounted to little more than a sink-or-swim ultimatum.

After graduating, he was drafted into the Korean War and assigned to serve in California for two years. There, he met a kindergarten teacher whom he would go on to marry. As I sat in their living room, I saw the two exchange quick smiles, a kind of grateful laugh to acknowledge their good fortune. Ms. Jones was born and raised in West Roxbury, and so the newly-weds moved back to the Boston area shortly after Mr. Jones completed his service. They settled in Cambridge, where Ms. Jones found a teaching job and Mr. Jones pursued his doctorate in philosophy, focusing on mathematical logic and computer programming. Doctorate in hand, Mr. Jones went on to put his programming expertise to work at a software engineering firm, where he stayed until his retirement a little over a decade ago. Soon after taking his job, he and his wife had the first of seven children. Photos of him and his children—all sixteen of them, including his seven children and nine grandchildren—lined the apartment.

Having vicariously learned about his life's journey through the keepsakes and picture frames around us, I then shifted the conversation towards his health. I had known Mr. Jones was diabetic, and so I had done a little reading beforehand. I learned that diagnosing diabetes in the elderly can be challenging. Its symptoms often arise gradually and are different from what is seen in younger patients. For instance, the tell-tale presence of glucose in the urine may be absent, and older diabetics have symptoms such as dry mouth and eyes, urinary incontinence, confusion, or fatigue. Since elderly patients may perceive such symptoms as benign, as nothing more than the bodily discomforts of growing old, they are often ignored. It comes as no surprise then that many cases of diabetes in older patients are only discovered after the vascular complications of the disease become apparent. Through conversations with Mr. Jones, I discovered that he squarely fell into that last group of elderly diabetics, those who receive a diagnosis of diabetes only after its complications have left their mark.

On a cold February day just a few years ago, Mr. Jones began to experience shortness of breath and a pain in his chest. Not wanting to worry his wife of nearly 50 years, he did his best to ignore the pain. But as time went on, the pain became less and less bearable. He finally informed his wife and the two decided to head to the nearest hospital. There, Mr. Jones was

THE SOUL OF A PATIENT

promptly diagnosed with an acute myocardial infarction, hospital lingo for what is colloquially known as a heart attack, and rushed into the cardiac catheterization lab. The cardiologist, Dr. Sampson, and his team quickly made an incision on Mr. Jones's inner thigh and inserted a catheter into his femoral artery. The team then threaded the guide wire against the flow of blood, up through the abdominal and thoracic aorta, and positioned it just upstream from the coronary arteries that supply the heart muscle with blood and oxygen. With the catheter in place, the team released repeated infusions of imaging dye to visualize Mr. Jones's coronary circulation.

The images that flickered across the adjacent monitor were not encouraging. The sinewy vascular tree, whose branches wrap around a healthy heart, was truncated. Mr. Jones had four separate blockages in his coronary arteries that were starving his heart muscle of oxygen and other vital nutrients. If blood flow was not effectively circumvented, these blockages would soon bring his heart, and ultimately his life, to end. As Mr. Jones lay on his back in the catheterization lab, his eyes and ears drowning in a sea of operating theater lights and voices, he overheard a member of the medical team utter the word "triple bypass." It turned out that two of the four blockages were in close proximity of one another, and blood could be rerouted around those two with a single bypass. This made the technical difficulty of the upcoming procedure only marginally easier, however. The medical team would still need to perform open-heart surgery to rewire the vasculature around his heart and create three new paths for blood flow, by borrowing segments of a healthy artery nearby.

The technical details of his upcoming procedure, of course, were not his most pressing concern. Mr. Jones was in pain. He was frightened by the possibility of leaving behind his family and, true to his reputation as an ever-protective husband and father, his mind immediately filled with practical advice he wished to relay to his daughter. There were financial loose ends—investment portfolios and bank account details—that he wanted her to tie up, so that he could leave his loved ones behind with a sense of financial security. Within moments, however, he realized that the window for that conversation had closed. His wife and children would have to navigate the practical—as well as the emotional and psychological—burden of his death without his guidance. It was, as he rightly recognized, out of his control.

Fortunately, Mr. Jones was in good hands. Dr. Sampson had performed over 3500 heart surgeries during the course of his career. Mr. Jones also had a couple others things going for him as well. His wife had brought him into the hospital early. The team that met him in the emergency room recognized the urgency of situation and acted accordingly. The necessary tests and labs were promptly ordered and performed, and Mr. Jones was transferred to a well-equipped surgical suite in which Dr. Sampson and his team were prepared to act quickly.

Mr. Jones went on to survive the day's events. He spent the next couple hours recovering in the white-walled interior of his hospital room with his wife and one of his daughters, Johanna. As he floated in and out of consciousness, he was immensely grateful that he would be able to continue caring for his family and, in due time, help them tie up those financial loose ends that had preoccupied him on the operating table. After Mr. Jones had regained some of his strength, his doctor took a seat by the bedside and explained to Mr. Jones what had happened. In addition to sharing details about the surgery, she informed him that one of the labs that were obtained when he first arrived at the hospital revealed that he had diabetes.

The diagnosis came as a surprise, but its timing made it seem incidental, something that registered as more of a blip on the radar screen instead of setting off alarm bells. As his doctor continued, however, Mr. Jones began to suspect that the diagnosis was more than a coincidence. Through subsequent conversations with his primary care physician and nurse practitioner, he came to appreciate the connection between diabetes and the threat that this posed to his health, He consulted his primary care physician to adjust his medications and diet. He kept meticulous track of his medicine schedule on a printed sheet of paper that could always be found on the coffee table next to his favorite chair. Since his time-tested system for staying on top of his medications was already in place, Mr. Jones had little trouble adding another medication into the mix to treat his diabetes.

As I reflected on my interactions with Mr. Jones over the past year, I realized that my sense of relief about his health was qualitatively different than it would have been had I just read over the same information in a patient's chart on the wards. It was not a difference of degree but rather a difference of kind. In many ways, Mr. Jones was the quintessential grandfather from family television sitcoms—warm, always ready with a story, and motivated by little else than his concern and sincere caring for family and friends. Coupled with the hospitality he showed in welcoming me into his home and our frequent conversations, I came to view him as a family member or close friend. I called him on holidays and his anniversary, and like a good friend, he would always ask me for updates on what I had mentioned in our last phone call or email exchange. Such a bond enhances the patient-doctor relationship on multiple levels. I imagine that it was something along these lines that prompted Dr. Francis W. Peabody to note in his address to an amphitheater of medical students that "one of the essential qualities of the clinician is interest in humanity. For the secret of the care of the patient is in caring for the patient."

One of the greatest insights I took away from my interactions with Mr. Jones, however, was that this has to be done conscientiously. Otherwise, it could compromise the judgment of a caregiver, by unconsciously making him or her less likely to make the tough decisions—for instance, delivering news likely to cause unnecessary worry or ordering a procedure unlikely to yield new information, but will most certainly inflict pain—that often go hand in hand with caring for patients. It was a lesson I came close to learning the hard way just a few short weeks later.

Every year, a week or two after Memorial Day, Mr. and Ms. Jones pack up their apartment and make their way north to their home in Maine for the summer. I had planned to swing by their apartment one last time before they left for the summer but, with the end of the academic year right around the corner, I became pressed for time and had to settle for a phone call. From his soft-spoken hello, I could tell that Mr. Jones had something heavy on his mind. Before I could ask, he filled me in on his stream of consciousness. He had been thinking about how limited his day-to-day activities had become, worried that his dependence on his wife only served to hold her back from her relatively active daily schedule.

"Lately I've been thinking about what would happen if Ms. Jones or I were to pass away," he said. "I really can't imagine life without her or any daily company. I'd probably remarry in a heartbeat. But I know that Ms. Jones would do the opposite. She's so active and I'm such a burden on her schedule." We talked a bit about the ways his health issues left him feeling disempowered. I was struck by the sadness in his tone. Although Mr. Jones did not appear to be suffering from depression, the reading I had glanced over prior to our initial meeting indicated that diabetic patients disproportionately suffer from depression. For instance, one in five elderly patients reportedly suffers from depression. That rate is double in diabetic patients.

Several times during the course of our conversation, he alluded to his inability to walk more than a hundred yards or so. "I think the farthest I've gotten in recent years is no more than

200 yards," he said. When I asked him to tell me more about what happens when he walks, something in his answer concerned me. It sounded as though he was experiencing shortness of breath upon exertion. I had shadowed a cardiologist for a few months two summers ago, and to me it sounded like a textbook presentation of cardiovascular disease—an elderly, obese man with a history of coronary artery disease who feels winded and short of breath when walking a few hundred feet.

Despite my concern, I didn't speak up. Later that night, I realized that my silence wasn't simply because I felt my clinical instincts as a first-year medical student were too limited to act. Instead, it was because I had come to view Mr. Jones as a close friend, one whom I didn't want to inconvenience unless it was absolutely necessary. I had learned about his shortness of breath just days before he left for his summer home in Maine. Moreover, I had learned about it right after it became clear to me that he was suffering from a certain frustration and loneliness about his immobility. The last thing I wanted to do was give him another reason to worry and force him to make a trip to the clinic, especially if that might provide no new insight or cause for concern.

Over the course of the next day or so, I grew increasingly worried. I became preoccupied by worst-case scenarios. What if I was right? What if Mr. Jones's heart health was in decline and he was just weeks away from another ischemic episode? Shouldn't I at least share my concern with either him or his primary care physician? Wasn't it, after all, better to be safe than sorry? And so, two days after Mr. Jones had mentioned his shortness of breath to me, I decided to get in touch with Dr. Rale. I relayed the pertinent parts of my phone conversation with Mr. Jones and mentioned that, although my clinical understanding was limited, I felt compelled to pass along what I had heard in case it warranted a closer look.

Dr. Rale and I followed up with Mr. Jones and, fortunately, it turned out to be nothing more than a miscommunication. There was, in the end, no reason for Mr. Jones to worry about his heart. However, the experience taught me an important lesson. I realized that truly caring for a patient as if he or she is a close friend is important, but that it must be done with an awareness of the ways in which such care can subtly make one shy away from inconveniencing a patient, even when it is clinically indicated.

My interactions with Mr. Jones also underscored the need to understand the array of issues—ranging from the biomedical to the psychosocial—that uniquely shape the care of a specific patient. By his own admission, Mr. Jones has a sedentary lifestyle. "My day doesn't consist of much nowadays. Ms. Jones takes care of the cooking and household work. She manages to do it despite her membership in four clubs here in the city, which meet regularly. That leaves me with my favorite chair, email, some reading, and our Netflix account," he said.

"I'm glad my wife is able to get out and about. It keeps her life interesting and I wish I could do the same," he once remarked. "Instead, my days often pass right here in the living room, with the occasional highlight of getting a glimpse of the rowers going by on the Charles." He then went on to describe the various permutations of rowers that occupy the Charles on a beautiful spring or summer day, underscoring just how much time he spends by the window in his apartment looking over the Charles.

When I asked what he felt kept him from having a more active lifestyle, he cited the pain in his lower back that he experiences when he walks. However, Dr. Rale had pointed out to that there were ways around that, ways to stay active and exercise despite his back pain. In fact, over the past few years, Dr. Rale has tried hard to coax Mr. Jones into exercising and losing weight. However, Dr. Rale had little success at getting

Mr. Jones to pursue a more active lifestyle, and despite his best efforts, Mr. Jones still showed little enthusiasm for exercise and weight loss.

While I was not responsible for treating Mr. Jones, I could not help but feel as though he was my first patient. As I had hoped, my interactions with him were formative from an educational standpoint and transformative from a personal one. I gave Mr. Jones a call to thank him again for welcoming me into his home and sharing his thoughts with me over the past year. I told him about how I was forever in his debt and felt as though it would be impossible to fully express my gratitude to him. In his ever-caring, ever-protective, ever-grandfatherly way, he managed to reply with a simple yet profound message. "I'm not sure if what I did deserves so much appreciation, but I'd be lying to you if I said there weren't several times in my own life when I felt grateful beyond words. On such occasions, I've realized that the best thing to do is to say thank you and then promise yourself to pay it forward. In your case, pay it forward by taking care of your future patients with the same sincerity, due diligence, and smile you showed me. If you do that, I assure you that we'll be more than even."

Invest in the Beginning

KIA BYRD

Growing up, I was rarely exposed to the "joys" of pregnancy. The youngest of three children, I never had the opportunity to watch my mother's belly swell; to hear her bark commands at my father to "run to the store" to satisfy her food cravings; to witness the communing of family and friends as my aunt welcomed guests to her extravagant and lavishly planned baby shower. I could only appreciate the stories—the stories about my mother that my older brothers would recount over and over at my request. At seven years old, still selfishly and egotistically obsessed with my own existence, I would inquisitively inquire, "What was it like when I was born?" Several years my senior, my brother would sit me on his lap, wrap his arms around me, in an almost paternal and protective manner, and describe to me the day of his eleventh birthday.

At the time, my father worked for the Jackson Public School District as the principal for one of Mississippi's only institutions for instruction in vocational education: The Career Development Center (CDC) of Jackson. Born in poverty-stricken, racially segregated Port Gibson, Mississippi, during the Civil Rights era, my father learned from an early age that absolutely nothing in life would be handed to him on a silver platter. One of nine children, my father would often recall summers during his childhood: grudgingly pulling himself from slumber at 5 a.m., complaining of the humid, stifling, southern mornings, as he accompanied his older male siblings around their modest home—tackling any handy work or laborious tasks that needed to be tended to during the day. In my father's recounts of his childhood, he would always mention how his own father instilled within him the essential values of manhood: hard work, integrity, and heritage. Born in Mound Bayou, Mississippi—the oldest U.S. all-Black municipality founded by ex-slaves, in

1887—my grandfather ensured that his family appreciated the legacy of hard work and self-determination inherent within the Black communities of Mississippi. Growing into adulthood and embodying the lessons from my grandfather, my father managed to work his way through both undergraduate and graduate school at two of Mississippi's most prominent historically Black institutions of higher education. Not bad for a young Black man in the South.

My mother grew up in a traditional household, a family of eight children headed by a strict patriarch. A country girl from Liberty, Mississippi, she would recall her early years—years when she would accompany her father on their family farm to feed pigs, raise chickens, and harvest the seasonal cucumbers, corn, berries, and nuts that sustained the family through the winter months. Relatively isolated from the hustling and bustling of the city, and molded by the values of a rural existence, my mother relied heavily on her mother and older sisters to serve as examples of Black femininity and womanhood. Proud Southern Belles in their own regard, the women of my mother's family upheld conventional values of the time: support for one's spouse, dedication to the family, care for one's appearance, and proper attention to one's demeanor and manner. Following high school, she developed an interest for business and finance. Realizing that her life was destined for more than Liberty could provide, she packed her belongings and headed for Jackson—"the Big City"—to pursue an education at a local business college. She would later find a career in banking, a career that would span over 20 years—not bad for a young Black woman from the country.

It was a Tuesday, a normal day in the Byrd household, as my father suited and prepared for his morning 8 a.m. commute. My mother, busy ironing clothes and preparing breakfast for my two brothers, had the day off from work. My eldest brother boarded a school bus and was whisked away to a summer enrichment day camp, while my older brother, anxiously anticipating his eleventh birthday festivities, stayed home with my mother. My brother described the day as "perfect"—an afternoon at the movie theater watching the latest Batman flick, lunch at his favorite Shoney's restaurant, an afternoon of pick-up basketball with his best friends, and, of course, chocolate ice cream birthday cake. "The day couldn't get any better." However, at around 5 o'clock that evening, the day took a turn.

My father returned home from work to find my mother complaining of intense abdominal pain. Two weeks prior, the family's obstetrician told my parents that the baby had the potential to come early, but unconvinced of an early delivery, my mother waited for the pain to subside and went about her normal activities. Approximately two hours later, she experienced a stronger, more intense wave of pain lasting a bit longer. Again, she waited for the pain to subside and went about her normal activities. Finally, at around 10:30 on that humid summer night, my father was convinced that "this baby's coming," and became determined to get my mother to the hospital as soon as possible. After quickly packing a bag for the hospital and nudging my mother and brother into his old 1982 Pontiac Bonneville, my father hit the gas pedal and made a dash for the hospital. After running two red lights and almost hitting a pedestrian on a bicycle, the family finally made it to Baptist Medical Center. My father grabbed the nearest wheelchair, rolled my mother into the delivery wing, and began filling out the necessary paperwork for the admissions clerk at the front desk. After a few minutes of waiting, my mother was taken to an examination room; however, minutes later, the physician announced that it was time to deliver. "I remember mama screaming," recalls my brother. "Then, I remember hearing your cries. I knew you had entered the world. The first time I saw you, I remember noticing your big eyes. You were so observant, as if everything was filled with wonder. It was the best belated birthday present I could have ever received."

In my family, children represent an abundance of possibility—the possibility to move and advance the family. Not only do they represent progression and forward movement, they come to symbolize an unbroken genealogy of Black experiences and resilience spanning the entirety of human history. Perhaps that explains why pregnancy has always represented, for me, a state shrouded in wonder, mystery, and awe—the awe of the unknown, of mystery, of possibility.

The sentiments held by members of my own family are representative of the sentiments felt by many African-Americans. The meaning of pregnancy is rooted in family and community. Pregnancy in the African-American community is a celebratory event, and an opportunity for ancestors and elders to transfer knowledge, history, tradition, and culture to a new generation. In addition, pregnancy provides an opportunity for community integration. The church is an important source for information and support. Consequently, the experience of pregnancy embodies a spiritual component, connecting a woman to her social community and more extensive spiritual community.

The African-American community possesses a variety of unique perspectives on the experience of childbirth, but the importance of culture to the experience of pregnancy is not unique to the experience of African-Americans. In traditional Nigerian culture, for example, new mothers are segregated from the family and community and later re-introduced into religious and socio-cultural structures. This stems from the ideology that seclusion equates protection and rest—a scenario that, according to the perspective of traditional Nigerian cultural beliefs, provides for better health outcomes for mother and baby. In India, pregnancy is considered a "blessing bestowed on young women," and being a mother is regarded as a socially significant and powerful role. Similar to the African-American traditions reflected during pregnancy, traditional Indian views of pregnancy acknowledge the necessity for support by elder women, extended family, and the community during the entire childbearing period. Regardless of the culture of origin, the responsibility of motherhood and experience of pregnancy represents a turning point of tremendous significance for women around the world.

My decision to enter medical school was one influenced by a multitude of factors. Above all, I genuinely desired to serve as a change-agent for communities like those in which I was raised, while also serving as a positive example for younger generations of black and brown youth around the globe. When I entered Harvard Medical School, I entered into a community of extraordinary individuals—a diverse community of students and expert clinicians of nearly every field. World-renowned scientists, researchers, physicians, and health policy experts taught my first-year courses; and I felt so fortunate to have the opportunity to learn medicine alongside some of the brightest and most capable people in the world—literally. But as the weeks and months of my first year rolled by, my attitude about my new environment began to change. I was consumed in a whirlwind of minutiae: molecular pathways, biochemical reactions, and cellular function. During my weekly patient clinics and Patient-Doctor I course, I rarely had the opportunity to interact with or learn from patients who looked like me. And on top of everything, I was running low on sleep, exercising less, and struggling to perfect the transition from college to medical school. I was unsatisfied with my experience and felt immensely removed from the populations whom I ultimately sought to serve. Had I made the right decision? Would my life's purpose be fulfilled in my work as a physician? Overwhelmed by self-doubt and uncertainty about the path that I had chosen, I sought opportunities that would reconnect me to my original perceptions of medicine, opportunities that would help to reaf-firm my decision to enter this noble and worthwhile profes-sion. Then, I found Medical Students Offering Maternal Support (MOMS).

MOMS is "a program that matches first-year medical stu-dents at Harvard with pregnant women at the Community Health Center, with the goal of empowerment through community partnership." I stumbled across the MOMS pro-gram and was immediately attracted to the program's purpose and goals, of encouraging students to advocate for patients, raising awareness around health disparities in birth outcomes, and providing longitudinal exposure to a unique patient population. MOMS represented the type of experience I desired for myself while at HMS, an opportunity to learn medicine from those members in the community, particularly women, who faced difficulties in accessing healthcare and means for social, political, and economic empowerment.

Around the same time, my sister-in-law announced that she was pregnant. I thought to myself, "How exciting! An op-portunity to find commonalities and similarities in the experi-ences of *two* women—my sister-in-law and soon-to-be "MOM" [MOMS patient]—as they embark on this journey of mother-hood!" However, the MOMS program would soon expose me to the stark realities and disparities in the antepartum experi-ences of my White sister-in-law from Rockville, Maryland, and my Black, Cape Verdean "MOM" from Dorchester, Massachusetts.

I met Darina on a Thursday afternoon in February. It was lunchtime at Harvard Medical School, and I had just suffered through an entire morning of small-group sessions and lec-tures. The "Integrated Human Physiology" course-block is, without question, the most difficult course within the first-year "New Pathways Curriculum," and my state of being at the time reflected such: I was operating on four hours of sleep, suffering from outrageous bright red pimples that had not reared their ugly heads since high school, and seriously doubting whether I had the necessary gumption and mental capacity to pass the upcoming physiology final—a four-hour beast that, according to the upperclassmen, was just as draining as it was difficult. I was scheduled to shadow in the OB/GYN department of the Community Health Center, and I was running behind. I immediately whipped out my iPhone to request an Uber: 6-minute wait—just enough time to grab one of those beef and bean burritos from Sami's, the food stand near Vanderbilt Residence Hall that I always frequented when I was in a rush. After a few minutes of impatient waiting, I quickly shoveled a few pieces of the beefy goodness into my mouth. A moment later, the Uber arrived, and I was off to the center.

When I arrived, I noticed that the Community Health Center looked quite distinct from many of the other clinics and Harvard-affiliated hospitals that I had visited. The most obvious difference: Nearly everyone in the clinic, at least everyone in the main lobby, was a minority—including the patients, security guards, and even the admissions clerks. The clinic was filled with a multitude of faces, all various shades of brown, and boisterous with the sounds of various languages that were all foreign to my ears. Upon entering, I approached the end of the admissions line, waiting for my turn at the front desk. When I finally reached the front of the line, a pleasant woman in a bright, green dress asked in a squeaky voice, "May I help you?" "Hi," I uttered awkwardly, "I'm a student at Harvard Medical School, and I'm here to shadow Dr. Sage." "She's expecting you. Follow me," she replied, as she slid back in her chair to stand. She led me around the corner and down a hallway lined with a series of black-and-white photographs, all depicting scenes from daily life in the Dorchester community. A thin and graceful Dr. Sage appeared. I remembered her blond hair and fair facial features from the first time I was introduced to her a few months prior.

After a brief conversation in her office, she informed me that there were a few new faces in the office, and perhaps, today would be the day that I would *finally* be assigned a patient for the MOMS program. Months had passed since I was promised a "mystery pregnant lady" to follow over the course of the academic year, and I was gradually losing confidence that I would have substantial time to follow my MOM over the remainder of the semester. Nevertheless, I shadowed Dr. Sage, visiting with the day's OB/GYN patients: watching as she conducted pap smears, asking typical first-year medical-student questions, and even palpating a few pregnant bellies with her guidance. I was thoroughly enjoying myself, but the clock was ticking. It was 5:30. Still no patient assignment.

By 6 o'clock, disappointment began to set in. Dr. Sage had excused herself, along with one of the OB/GYN interns, to perform an endometrial biopsy. I was left to entertain myself. After twiddling my thumbs for what seemed like an eternity, and attempting to read a few pages of notes for the next day's physiology lectures, Dr. Sage entered the office. She had found a patient. I immediately perked up and asked when I would have the opportunity to meet her. "Right now. Come on," Dr. Sage beckoned. At that moment, the knots began to form in my stomach. The palms of my hands began to sweat. I was nervous. I couldn't believe it. I thought to myself, "I'm a confident person. I can hold pretty decent conversations. I have a pretty easy-going personality." So why was I so apprehensive? Would the mystery pregnant lady like me? Would she ask me "medical" questions to which I had no idea how to respond? Would she feel comfortable with me? Would she trust me? I suppose most medical students, and even many physicians, ask themselves the very same question before meeting a new patient: Will I demonstrate the ability to connect?

One of the most important lessons that I have learned from patient encounters, during my first year of medical school, is the fact that first impressions are often the most critical moments in the patient-doctor (in-training) relationship. Vocal tone, eye contact, and even small gestures have the ability to influence how well a physician demonstrates the ability to relate to patients. It is especially important to establishing rapport quickly with a new patient. Although this patient encounter, in the examination rooms of the Health Center, would be somewhat different from the typical patient interviews that I was accustomed to in my "Patient-Doctor I" course at HMS, I was determined to ensure a good beginning to my relationship with the mystery pregnant lady.

When we finally arrived at her door, Dr. Sage knocked and we entered. "Good evening, Darina. This is Kia, your Harvard medical student from the MOMS program. Kia, this is Darina." As Dr. Sage finished the introductions, I walked towards Darina and extended my hand to shake hers. As she reached over to place her hand in mine, I noticed that her face, of a caramel complexion, appeared rather youthful, almost as youthful as my own. "How old was she?" I thought. In my mind, I immediately characterized her as mid-to-late twenties. What did she do for a living? What was her family like? Dr. Sage then proceeded to explain a bit more about the MOMS program—detailing logistics and explaining my role as a "medical student offering maternal support." I watched Darina as she listened attentively to Dr. Sage, her dark, curly hair bouncing loosely as she nodded her head in understanding. When Dr. Sage finally finished the explanation and all consent forms were signed, she finally left Darina and me to have a private conversation. After the door closed, a few seconds of uncomfortable silence passed. Realizing that the conversation was not going to start itself, I thought that it was only appropriate that I begin with a few words about myself. A first year medical student who was inconveniently inserting herself into the life of a first time mother, I felt that it was only logical that she find out a bit about me first. I told her that I was born in Mississippi, talked a little about growing up in the South, mentioned that I lived in DC for a few years to attend Howard University before coming to medical school, and explained to her my motivations for pursuing medicine and, potentially, a future as an obstetrician. "Darina, tell me a little about yourself."

Darina is a healthy 22-year-old woman who was born in Boston and lived the entirety of her life thus far in Dorchester, Massachusetts. The daughter of immigrants from Cape Verde—an island in the central Atlantic Ocean off the coast of West Africa—Darina described the importance of growing up in the diversity of the Dorchester community. A resident of Upham's Corner, which contains the largest concentration of people of Cape Verdean origin in Boston, Darina was raised speaking both English and Cape Verdean Creole, a blend of Portuguese and African languages preserved by African slaves en route to the Americas during the 16th century. Fascinated by the various cultures of the African Diaspora, I asked her how she "identified" within the context of living as an American. She explained to me that although she identifies with the experiences of African-Americans, she is distinctly Cape Verdean—a cultural experience that cannot be encompassed by the usage of terms such as "Black" or "African-American." After graduating from high school, Darina decided not to attend college and chose, instead, to enter the workforce. An employee for a Boston transportation company, she expressed that she enjoyed her job. "The people are really friendly, and my work is essentially at a desk. I guess that's a good thing, since I'll need to stay off my feet, huh?" she laughed. "I guess so," I chuckled in reply. The conversation seemed to be going well, and I felt genuinely excited about the forthcoming opportunity to learn more about and from a fellow sister of the African Diaspora.

ACCEPTANCE

After a while, I heard a knock at the examination room door and Dr. Sage re-entered. "Well, I have the date and time for your next appointment scheduled," she announced. "Is there anything else that you need from me or any other questions that you may have?" Darina shook her head and stood up from her chair to leave. We quickly exchanged contact information, typing expeditiously on the screens of our iPhones, and finally bid our farewells and "see you laters." As I packed my belongings to leave the clinic, Dr. Sage asked, "So. What do you think?" "Seems like a good fit," I responded with a smile. I felt comfortable with Darina and could only hope that she felt the same about me. As I waved goodbye to the security guard and stepped outside of the clinic to locate my return Uber, a million thoughts and questions were running through my head. It had finally occurred to me that Darina was my age. I couldn't fathom the responsibility of caring for a child at 22. At this point in my life, I was still learning to cook without setting the stove on fire. What would my life be like if I were pregnant? Was Darina scared? Was she nervous? As I traveled back to Longwood, I pondered these questions and my brief conversation with the Cape Verdean American "mystery pregnant lady," who would teach me so much about society and myself.

Several weeks rolled by before I had the opportunity to see Darina again. We communicated on a weekly basis via text messaging, but we never voiced concerns or suggestions over anything substantial—at least from my perspective. I would often shoot her a message and ask, "How's it going?" In reply, I would never receive more than a simple, "Good" or "Everything is going fine." At the time, I was in the midst of our final and lengthiest course of first year, "Immunology, Microbiology, and Pathology," and I had just completed a stressful, yet rewarding, stint as Co-Director for our HMS first-year cultural exposition, "FABRIC." During those weeks of limited contact with my MOM, I felt extremely disappointed in myself for not maintaining more extensive contact with Darina. I felt selfish for failing to make more of a concerted effort to *really* get to know Darina. I vowed to establish a more consistent and substantial relationship with my MOM over the remainder of the semester. Her upcoming ultrasound appointment, an appointment at which the full fetal survey would be conducted, would be my next opportunity to do so.

The night before the full fetal ultrasound, I received an unexpected phone call from Darina around 8:30 p.m., and I was just finishing up a few flashcards from the day's lectures when I answered the phone. Somewhat surprised, as this was the first time she had ever called me, I actually expected the worst. Was she injured? Had something gone wrong with the baby? "Darina, how are you? Is everything ok?" I hoped that my voice had not alarmed her. "I'm fine," she replied. "I just wanted to remind you of my appointment tomorrow." I expressed to her that the appointment was on my schedule and that I would be present. From her phone call, however, I sensed that there were other things on her mind. She had not called merely to remind me of her appointment; she wanted to talk. After a few moments of pleasantries and small talk, I finally asked: "So, how are you feeling about tomorrow?" Just the simple question alone was enough to spur a 30-minute conversation. Although filled with excitement at the opportunity to become more familiar with her baby's anatomy and to finally discover the baby's sex, she expressed an understandable sense of angst in anticipation of the next day's appointment. She mentioned that her entire family hoped for a baby girl. Dolls had been purchased: "It's a Girl" baby bibs had been wrapped and gifted, and small, bright pink dresses had been acquired. I thought to myself, "Wow. There's so much pressure on her to have a girl. What if her baby is a boy?" Regardless, I reassured her that whatever the baby's sex, he or she would be just as beautiful as Darina. She giggled. And after expressing so much thanks and gratitude, she wished me a good evening, and ended the call. I must admit that after our conversation, I began to feel a bit nervous myself. "Silly, Kia," I thought. I wasn't even a member of her family. I had no reason to be nervous. Nevertheless, that same night, I slept and dreamt of Darina and her unborn baby.

The OBs at the health center had scheduled Darina's ultrasound appointment to take place at the hospital. Luckily, the walk was only a few blocks. A few days prior, Darina informed me that I should meet her there. I had only been to the hospital twice, but I was confident that I could find my way without assistance. Roaming aimlessly, I found the nearest set of elevators and took them to the seventh floor. Piece of cake. When I stepped off of the elevator, I read a set of double doors that read "Cardiovascular Medicine." I knew immediately that this was *not* where I would find Darina. I glanced at my phone for the time: 2:43. I was going to be late. I scurried back to the elevator and returned to the lobby area. There, I approached the staff at the Welcome Desk and asked for directions to the Maternal and Fetal Medicine Department. After commenting that the entire hospital was "one big maze," she equipped me with a map of the medical center and sent me on my way to search for Darina.

When I finally arrived at the correct waiting room, it was 2:50. I scanned the waiting room, hoping that she had not already been called. "Kia!" I heard a voice shout from behind me. I turned around to find Darina sitting with two other women whom I had never seen before. As I walked towards them, Darina stood, greeted me with a warm embrace, and introduced me to the two women—her older cousins—who accompanied her. They both possessed a similar caramel complexion to Darina's, and, looking at them collectively from a distance, anyone would have guessed that they were sisters. Darina's cousins were both a year older, both had children, and both lived within a two-mile radius from her. Needless to say, they were extremely close, and considered themselves each other's primary means of social support. As we waited for Darina's name to be called, we conversed about popular culture: movies, music, and the "happening" spots in Boston. I was surprised that we enjoyed so many similar things. In fact, for the duration of nearly the entire waiting period, we all participated in a spirited debate about who was the better and more socially conscious rapper of our generation: Kendrick Lamar or J. Cole. I was amused, and as I laughed at the elements of our shared culture, observing Darina and each of her cousins at a time, I noticed something that forced me to double take: bruises—multiple, discolored patches of skin; two or three on the faces of each of her cousins. My thoughts were immediate: domestic violence. Had they been abused? Had Darina suffered from similar circumstances? What did this mean for her and her baby? Forcing myself to refrain from drawing unnecessary conclusions, I quickly suppressed the thoughts—though never removing them too far from the front of my mind. The nurse finally called Darina, and we all accompanied her to the examination room.

To say the least, Darina's baby was perfect. As the ultrasound technician examined the fetus and the approximate measurements of its anatomical structures, she commented that the baby appeared to be developing well—right smackdab in the middle of his or her growth curve. The entire occasion became much more than an opportunity to observe a full fetal survey and ultrasound, however. It became an opportunity for me to observe Darina in her element, an opportunity to see how she related and interacted within the social structure of her family. It became an occasion for celebration and laughter, a celebration of life and motherhood. Approximately 45 minutes into the appointment, the technician finally revealed what we had all been waiting for: the baby's sex. Watching the ultrasound screen, we stared at the tiny structure between the baby's legs. Darina leaned towards me and asked me to confirm what we were all seeing. Indeed, we were all staring at the genitalia of Darina's unborn baby boy. Filled with excitement and joy, a cacophony of sounds filled the examination room. Eager to share the news, the three cousins immediately posted photos to Instagram, authored messages for Facebook, and sent text messages to family and friends. Everyone was eager to share Darina's good news: a sweet, precious baby boy would be entering the world. I guessed that it was time to return those pink "It's a Girl" baby bibs.

After leaving the hospital, we decided to converse over dinner at a nearby food court a few blocks from the medical center. Apparently, I was somewhat of a mystery to Darina's family, and her cousins were curious of my motivations for serving as their younger cousin's "medical student offering maternal support." I explained my desire to work with and advocate for minority women, and, potentially, for a future career as an OB/GYN after completing medical school and residency. They wanted to know about my family, where I grew up, what I did for fun in the city, where I went to school, how I got into Harvard, and even if I had a significant other. I felt overwhelmed by their questions. Was it my place to reveal so much about myself?

After surviving their collective interrogation, I asked how they were getting home. There was no one designated to drive them back to Dorchester, and I highly doubted that any of them had a car. Darina informed me that they had taken the bus to the hospital and would be taking the same route home. Darina had taken off from work that day to make her appointment. It had taken her an hour-and-a- half to travel by bus, and would take her another two hours to return home in 5 o'clock traffic. I asked about her home environment. She lived with her mother, only a few blocks from her grandmother and cousins. Her mother worked to support herself, as Darina's father remained in Cape Verde and lacked the ability to support the family financially. Her mother was managing a variety of chronic diseases, and Darina admitted the difficulty in watching her mother's declining health, as she, herself, grappled with the idea of caring for a new baby in a few months. I asked about her baby's father. Would he be around to help care for the baby? Was he providing financial support? Her boyfriend resided in Mission Hill, and although they maintained frequent communication, a lack of reliable transportation hindered them from seeing each other on a regular basis. She spoke highly of her boyfriend, but left me with an uncomfortable feeling that, ultimately, Darina would bear the overwhelming burden of caring for her child alone.

We finished dinner, and after exchanging hugs and goodbyes, the three cousins boarded the city bus to return home to Dorchester. On my walk home, I pondered the various challenges that Darina would face in the coming months: raising a child as an unwed mother, lacking transportation and flexibility to attend postnatal appointments, and working to support both her mother's health expenses and her new baby boy. I also recalled the multiple bruises on the faces of her cousins. Was Darina returning to a violent home or community environment? I immediately thought of my pregnant sister-in-law, whose "clinical picture" was such a stark juxtaposition to that of Darina. My sister-in-law—a 33-year-old woman of Czechoslovakian descent, who presented to her OB/GYN at six weeks' gestation. She had recently celebrated her five-year wedding anniversary, worked as an RN with a Bachelor's Degree in nursing, and lived in a relatively safe community. She was looking forward to her second pregnancy, the first of which resulted in a beautiful, healthy baby boy—now three years of age. Although her pregnancy did not come without the stresses of caring for another human being, she was well-supported by a husband who was present and involved throughout the entire pregnancy, a mother who helped with cooking and child-care, and a job that allowed her time off and flexibility during the perinatal period. She did not come home to an environment where there was a question of domestic violence. She did not face the uncertainty that she would possibly have to raise her child alone. And though I am immensely grateful for the health and success of her pregnancy, I often wonder if the outcomes for her and my niece would have been different if she resided in another part of the city; if she did not have a substantial education or medical background; if she had a darker complexion.

Many Black mothers, like Darina, across the nation face similar situations; and, in many instances, circumstances surrounding issues of race, poverty, and socioeconomic factors have a substantial impact on birth outcomes for these populations of women. In the United States, infants born to mothers of African descent are more than twice as likely to die during the first year of life as infants born to mothers of European descent. Other adverse birth outcomes that are disproportionately more prevalent in African-American communities include low birth-weight and preterm delivery, which are also major causes of cerebral palsy, developmental delays, and vision and hearing impairments. Potential explanations for the disparate rates of adverse birth outcomes among African-Americans and European-Americans include socioeconomic differences and stress. A number of social factors are associated with adverse birth outcomes, including poverty, inadequate access to health care and insurance, limited education, and poor health behavior. In addition, African-American women more commonly experience social disadvantages, such as single parenthood and poverty. Stressors such as living in a low income and low-resourced community with higher levels of crime or violence, and racial discrimination may also contribute to ethnic disparities in adverse birth outcomes. Many African-American women are both mother and breadwinner. Consequently, it becomes important that social and community support, similar to the MOMS program, be made available for mothers of African descent, like Darina, in an effort to contribute to more positive health for both mother and baby.

Darina was now 30 weeks, and this would be one of the last opportunities for me to attend one of her prenatal appointments before the end of the HMS academic year. I arrived at the Community Health Center on a Monday evening a few minutes earlier than Darina's scheduled 5:40 p.m. appointment. Darina arrived a few moments later, checked in, and followed me into the waiting room. We sat down in a pair of the clinic's standard turquoise-blue waiting chairs and exchanged greetings. She had just gotten off work and was, understandably, fatigued. After catching her breath for a few moments, she updated me on her last appointment, one that I had unfortunately missed because of a class. She mentioned that she had been administered a blood glucose test; everything was normal and her pregnancy was progressing as planned. She also seemed somewhat shocked that the typical "symptoms" of pregnancy that her cousins and older female family members warned her about were non-existent for her. She had no food cravings, no morning sickness, no leg swelling. After months of debate and discussion with her family, she had also decided on a name for her baby boy. His name would take on the first letter of his father's first name, a four-generation tradition that Darina felt compelled to pass on to her unborn child. She was sailing, seemingly unaffected by the stereotypical physical and emotional manifestations of carrying another human being.

"I love being pregnant, and I love my baby," she declared, "but sometimes it can be so annoying." "What do you mean?" I asked, unsure of how to approach a statement of such ambiguity. It was finally summer. The days were sunny; the nights were warm; the summer festivities were heating up; the girls were sporting cut-off shorts and belly rings; and Darina was missing out. Her cousins and friends would call every weekend, raving about their latest adventures "out on the town," the previous evening's concerts, or their most recent trips to Revere Beach—and all that she could do was listen. "I can't fit into any of my cute clothes, and it's so obvious, everywhere that I go, that I'm pregnant. It's so frustrating," she pouted. Standing on her feet for extended periods of time was becoming more and more difficult, and she expressed sentiments of what I perceived to be resentment. She appeared restricted and inhibited—like a young bird, eager to fly but forced into submission by the invisible constraints of life and responsibility. This was the first time that I had heard her speak of such things. "Have you spoken to anyone else about how you're feeling?" I asked. She explained to me that, according to the elders of her family and culture, it was considered selfish to complain of such "trivial" things. A baby was a blessing, and she refused to express these sentiments to her family. "I know that I'll get over it eventually, but I just don't feel like myself." It seemed that as Darina's newly-named and rapidly developing baby boy was developing an identity of his own, Darina seemed to be losing her own in the process.

After her appointment, I sat with Darina and asked about her concerns going forward. She relayed to me her resentment towards her boyfriend, whom she described as far removed from the entire childbearing experience. "He doesn't *have* to come to these appointments. He doesn't *have* to stop seeing his friends. I've felt helpless throughout this entire process." Her eyes filled with tears, and I knew in that moment that I was likely the only person she had voiced this to. I was not a member of her family, but in being somewhat removed from her day-to-day existence, I could see that she trusted me enough, even as a non-relative, to keep that information safe.

And I loved acting as her personal counselor and advisor—recommending social support groups and hospital mental health services that could help her more than I could. I enjoyed our personal connection and felt empowered by the idea that I could play some role in empowering *her*. Trained in providing information that could be helpful for mothers at all stages of pregnancy, I showered her with information, ideas, and questions to potentially ask her OB/GYN during her next visit. I encouraged her to always be an advocate for herself, as the health of her baby and that of her own life and well-being were just as much her responsibility as that of the physicians who cared for her. I wanted her to feel powerful—to feel active in the decision-making process regarding her pregnancy. I hoped that I could give her the tools—at least some of them—to ensure that she never felt helpless. And, as overly-ambitious as I was as a first-year Harvard medical student, I walked away from Darina that evening, inspired to always provide my future patients with the education and resources that they needed to make informed decisions about their own healthcare.

The weeks rolled by, and as the summer ended and the new school year approached, I once again transformed into the neurotic medical student: throwing myself into my school work, sleeping less, and obsessing over abstracts and papers for upcoming conferences. It was the middle of September, and the second-year medical students were already immersed in the details of the human nervous system. One night, while finishing up an assignment for the next day's tutorial, my mind wandered to Darina. How was her baby? How was she? I wanted to call her to check in and to see how life was progressing for her. At the same time, I felt guilty for waiting this long to reach out to her. I had missed her delivery due to an international research trip, and I was reluctant to even contact her. Letting my insecurities get the best of me, I decided to forego the phone call. Nevertheless, Darina and her baby boy stayed on my mind for the next week. I ultimately made the decision to pick up the phone.

As the phone rang, I grew anxious. What if she didn't answer? Part of me actually hoped that my call would go to voicemail, but part of me also hoped that she would respond. After a few moments, I finally heard her boisterous, high-pitched voice. "Kia! How are you, dear?" I was relieved. We spent the next 40 minutes catching up on the joys of her life as a new mother. She told me about the sleepless nights, the difficulties of breast feeding, the pride she felt whenever someone exclaimed, "He looks just like you!" She wanted to tell it all. And I owed her the opportunity to tell it all.

Similar to my commitment to invest in the beginning of our relationship with honesty and openness, investing in the end of our visits with purposeful reflection and establishing mutual understanding became my goal for our final conversation. I asked about her hopes for the future and her dreams for herself and for her child. Darina thought for a moment. She finally stated that she simply prayed for the safety and protection of her family as they lived, struggled, and laughed day-to-day.

She held no expectations, and her words lingered with me. No one is certain of their life's course over the next year, month, day, or even the next hour. The only moment that is certain is the present, and Darina conveyed that message to me. As we said our goodbyes, she thanked me for all of my help and dedication to her family over the past several months. But as I hung up the phone, I reflected on how much she, in turn, had taught me about my future role as a physician and the part that I have to play, even as a medical student, in advocacy and leadership for the communities that I serve.

The experience of participating in the MOMS program and having the opportunity to learn medicine from minority patients has provided me with a renewed sense of purpose in medicine, and a renewed perspective by which I hope to approach medical education. Entering into this experience, I possessed a rather vague idea of how I sought to practice medicine. My knowledge of what constituted a good physician was loosely based on the limited interactions that I held with the handful of physicians I had encountered and shadowed during my undergraduate experiences, but I lacked a clear and substantial understanding of what a physician *actually* does.

Physicians are perceived as experts—as nearly superhuman—as we are expected to think, to know, and to do without hesitation. Society looks to us because we have the answers. But what happens when we don't? Operating within the culture of a profession that prioritizes knowledge over curiosity, the MOMS program allowed me the opportunity to ask questions and initiate conversations, not to elicit information in fulfillment of a task or for evaluation, but in genuine interest for the concerns, thoughts, and experiences of the patient.

At the beginning of my interactions with Darina, she expected that I, the medical student from Harvard Medical School, would hold the answers to her inquiries and requests. However, over the course of the past few months, Darina would become *my* instructor, as impactful in my life and medical education as any Harvard Medical School professor or clinician. She introduced me to the principles of establishing a trusting patient-doctor relationship: engaging shared experiences, attuning to the needs and perceptions of the patient, and viewing the patient, not merely as a collection of isolated organ systems, but as a holistic culmination of experiences, beliefs, values, and traditions in human form.

My experiences as a participant in the MOMS program have further reaffirmed my decision to utilize my career as a platform for the advocacy of underserved and disadvantaged women of color. As physicians and physicians-in-training, we must not view our practices in isolation, but as individual components of a larger social and political structure that impacts the lives of entire populations of individuals. As an African-American medical student, I am committed to utilizing my training in medicine for the promotion of more equitable and better quality healthcare for patients of minority and disadvantaged backgrounds. Accomplishing this task requires embracing an ideology that integrates medicine with community beliefs and values, economics, and politics, while advocating for the well-being of those disadvantaged by social systems. Darina, thank you for influencing my own definition of what it means to uphold the principles of patient-centered healthcare and what it means to serve the world as a physician.

Like a Job

ALEKS OLSZEWSKI

Bradley is from the Boston area, one of 14 children. His parents and many of his siblings still live nearby in the city. When Bradley was 6 months old, his mother signed him up for the Metropolitan Council for Educational Opportunity (METCO) list, which gave inner-city children the opportunity to attend school in the suburbs. The waiting list was long, but she put all of her children on it as soon as they were born, to increase their chances of a good education away from the negative influences of the schools in their own neighborhoods. By the seventh grade, Bradley was transferred to the suburbs for school. Without this change, he feels confident he would be "dead like all of my neighborhood friends." His best friend died in high school. "I've seen a lot, and now with this disease, I feel like I've gone through everything." He was studious, he played sports, and he was involved. His friends from the neighborhood sold crack cocaine and tried to get him to do so as well. He tells me they ridiculed him, but he never tried it. 'They told me I was lame. I told them, 'no I'm just smart.' Now, I'm the only one alive."

Bradley didn't fully fit in with his friends back home, but he also struggled at his new, predominantly white, wealthy school. However, when he talks about this, it is almost as an aside. He knows that transitioning to such a different school should be stressful and difficult. But meeting Bradley, it wouldn't be hard to believe that he transitioned and made friends easily. He has a way of making you feel at ease in any situation. His stories are enrapturing and emotional. His sense of humor is sarcastic and deadpan; whenever a conversation turns uncomfortable and you have no idea what to say, Bradley throws in a perfect one-liner, with a giant grin. And the conversation flows easily again.

In college, Bradley studied pediatric psychology. He loved school but when his girlfriend got pregnant his third year, he dropped out and started working at a juvenile detention center to support his family. At first, he was terrified to work there. "I didn't want to be around those kids. I was scared! I acted like I wasn't, but I was!" When asked about some of the more difficult aspects of his job, he looks away and says bluntly, "I saw terrible things. I had to do terrible things. It's like what you see on TV." Then he changes the subject.

One of his first days at work, he was called in to break up a fight. By the time he got there, one of the boys was beaten up so badly he was having trouble breathing. They called 911, but by the time the ambulance arrived, it was too late. The boy had passed away. The emotional strain of Bradley's job was matched by physical stress. The hours were long and brutal, and he was always on his feet. He often worked 3 a.m. to 11 a.m. After he became a supervisor, he found himself often tired, and he became less active outside of the workplace. At the same time, his eating habits deteriorated, as he started ordering out with his coworkers every night.

One night, some of the boys got into a fight. It escalated, and Bradley had to handcuff one boy and secure him to the floor, something he had done countless times before. But this time was different. For some reason, he lost his strength. He worked a double shift the next day, with his second shift from 3 a.m. to 7 a.m. He still didn't feel well that night, so when he came home he made a doctor's appointment. He felt a general pain and weakness in his muscles. These were symptoms that he had been experiencing and ignoring intermittently for about a year. But they had never scared him like this before; this was the first time he was literally unable to do a task he used to consider easy. He called the doctor's office, but was feeling better when his appointment came around, so he cancelled it and ignored his slowly progressing symptoms.

Three months later, he felt worse than he had since the incident that alarmed him, and he left work early, around 10 a.m., to go to the clinic and see what might be wrong. At the clinic, they found that his blood pressure was 200/100, a hypertensive crisis. Everything hurt. He was transferred to the ER in an ambulance and was admitted. Two weeks later, he was still in the hospital. His blood tests showed that his kidneys were "functioning like a 90-year-old man," he recalled them saying to him. He continued to feel weak, "like my muscles weren't working." He was initially diagnosed with a heart attack, but Bradley's recurring chest pains and episodes of muscle weakness kept bringing him back to the hospital. In and out of the hospital, he was often calling in to take off from work. He eventually used up all of his vacation days. "I wasn't feeling like I was getting any better." Repeated episodes of muscle weakness started pointing to a non-cardiac etiology, and a diagnosis was made of polymyositis, or chronic inflammation of his muscles. Testing for this, however, was negative—officially defining him as a mystery patient. "Everyone was confused. They went back and forth about it being a heart attack or not. Everything was up in the air, and it seemed like no one knew what was going on. I was getting scared." Bradley was passed from team to team. He was gawked at, squinted at, asked the same questions over and over again. With every return visit, the new attending glanced at his papers and read, "So, you have a history of a heart attack, does this resemble those symptoms?" He would try to explain that the heart attack was a misdiagnosis, but the note remained unchanged.

His episodes always started with chest pain on his right side, which then spread to the left. His third time going in for one of these episodes, he also felt like he had a cold. X-rays showed a fluid build-up in his chest and swelling in his right leg. He explained, "Fluid started leaking out of my pores, my leg was so swollen. They told me it was fluid around my heart, caused by the steroids. I freaked out. It was tough because I was taking so much of it. I was immune to a certain amount of prednisone, which made me feel like an addict. I couldn't walk or do anything without high doses of it; and I don't even believe in meds. It took a huge toll on me, mentally. It was the only thing that made my muscles feel better. No one told me that it's going to help you but it's going to kill you at the same time. I had no idea." With steroids, a common side effect is swelling or edema, and, in Bradley's case, the swelling led to fluid leakage through his skin.

Bradley's steroid dose was tapered off to help his edema, and he tried various pain medications. Only morphine worked. But he struggled to take it because it made him feel nauseated and "goofy." No one discussed the side effects and precautions for steroid or morphine use. Instead, he was told, "Just take this, it'll make you feel better." There was a great deal of miscommunication. Bradley felt more like a teaching tool than a patient. His team didn't seem to be interested in explaining things to Bradley. They were interested in solving the mystery. "I guess I had a team of doctors, but they all didn't talk to each other. They were trying to solve it themselves, telling me, 'You're a rare gem in this hospital.' They all came to see me, taking pictures. I didn't want everybody showing me off. I'm just worried that I'm going to die, and here they are, telling me I'm intriguing." But he ends this angry description with an incredibly mature and selfless reflection: "After thinking about it for a while, I didn't mind. I was, like, if this is going to help the next person, go for it. Do whatever you need."

However, Bradley was infuriated by the tone and nature of the interview questions with every visit. "They kept asking me, 'Do you do any drugs? Are you an avid cocaine user?' I was getting pissed. Listen man, I don't do any of that stuff. Why do you keep asking me? Are you asking me that because I'm Black? Every doctor asked me the same thing. Like I said, the docs didn't talk to each other." And still no diagnosis was made, no explanations were given. "At that point, I didn't know what was going to happen to me," he said. "I had this pain in my chest, and I am thinking, 'What the hell is going on with me?' It felt like my heart was skipping beats." The medical teams working with Bradley failed to draw any conclusions from interviewing him, and they mistrusted his stories at the same time, implying he was somehow at fault.

His medical care seemed to encompass all of the stereotypical healthcare failures we discuss as first year medical students. His care was fragmented and his teams did not communicate. He was treated as a spectacle rather than as a patient. He felt that he served as a teaching tool, but that his care team had no interest in teaching or helping *him*. His care team did not trust him when he corrected them or denied drug abuse. He felt that racial stereotypes were influencing the way clinicians treated and questioned him. When mistakes were made in diagnosis and note taking, no apology was offered. No explanation was provided for why multiple misdiagnoses were made or why the tests that proved them wrong were not done sooner. Side effects and contraindications were not made clear to him. Not a single clinician seemed capable of stopping to place himself in Bradley's shoes or considering this terrifying experience from a patient's perspective.

Hearing directly from Bradley, rather than reading or talking about his case abstractly in class, has helped me to cement in my mind the ways that medical care fails to help patients, and hopefully has made me acutely aware of these giant problems that are common issues patients encounter. These are flaws in healthcare at both the systems level and the individual level. Hearing about Bradley's experience certainly reminds me about the *why* in the constant discussion of improving patient care at the systems and individual levels, but it also provides me with the *how*—how things can go wrong—to help steer me in the right direction in my future as a healthcare provider.

Finally, things came together. Bradley saw a rheumatologist who ordered a muscle biopsy and confirmed that he had systemic lupus erythromatosus (SLE or "lupus"), as the cause of the symptoms. Lupus is a disease of the body's immune system, when the body attacks your own tissues and organs. The day Bradley learned his diagnosis was the day that "everything started." While on his cocktail of steroids and other immunosuppressive medications, the side effects were unbearable for him. Despite being in a great deal of pain, he rarely took his pain medications because he hated the way they made him feel. At one point, he was taking 30 pills in the morning, and some he had to take a second time each day. "I hate taking pills. I was pissed off and I was, like, 'I'm not taking this stuff no more.' I was feeling better, I believe, when I was not taking some of those pills. I told the docs I took them, but I lied."

"A lot of the drugs made me sicker than I was," he lamented. He vomited many times a day while on steroids. He carried a bag with him at all times, and his kids knew to be ready to help him if he felt the need to vomit. "They were helpful, but I didn't want them to see me like that. Not to be nasty, but the bag was scented. It was disgusting." Bradley didn't completely neglect his medications, but randomly "took days off from it." "The worst was my kids seeing me throw up," he said. Bradley knew that he could cover up the pain symptoms in front of his children, but the vomiting was impossible to hide. So he chose pain.

Bradley was worried about what his kids' friends would think of him, about appearing to be a weak and needy dad. He was used to supporting his family since he was a child. So Bradley took control of his condition in his own way. "I started to have flare-ups, but I wouldn't go in. I would just sit, and I learned how to meditate the pain away." No one taught Bradley any pain management techniques. He trained himself.

At face value, Bradley may appear to be a noncompliant patient. He often did not take his meds. However, he repeatedly tells me that he is "just trying to get better. I am in it to win it." So his goals certainly match those of his physicians. To understand his noncompliance, one must ask "*Why* are you trying to get better?" and the loud and clear answer to this is "For my family." Along this vein, "*Why* are you noncompliant?" And the answer is simple and logical: because the side effects of the medication are more debilitating and more embarrassing in front of his family than are the disease symptoms.

Losing his ability to do any of the activities he enjoyed, along with his opportunity to support his family, Bradley felt that he lost his identity. His life seemed out of his control. Most stressfully, money became a problem. Bradley is engaged with three children. He has two children with his fiancé, Rhonda, plus another son who lives with Bradley's previous wife. For a while, he lived off of his pension and benefits, but that only lasted two years. He is now being supported by his fiancé and earnings from "the occasional paper my son delivers." He went from "top-notch" health insurance to MassHealth (Medicaid). Not used to such financial difficulties, he describes his lowest point as the month when he couldn't afford the copays on his prescriptions. "They treat you so different when you can't afford medications. I felt so poor. We had to apply for food stamps. I've never done that before." His household income went from $53,000 to $8,000 a year, as he watched his plans for a wedding and a house go on the back burner. "I would come home from the hospital again, sit in my living room when no one was there and cry. I don't think I would ever do it, but it often crossed my mind, "What would happen if I just wasn't here? It did cross my mind. I can't go back to work; I feel useless. What am I supposed to do?"

ACCEPTANCE

With time to adapt, Bradley once again finds himself experiencing joy in the little things, cracking jokes during football games with his extended family, and playing with his children. Through his self-therapy and thanks to support from his family, Bradley has come to realize that he still has a purpose. Having had a few years to come to terms with his inability to support his family financially, Bradley sees the time he has as an opportunity to become close with his kids. He is an incredibly attentive stay-at-home dad.

One day, I went to the doctor with Bradley and his daughter Audrey, who was suffering unbearable ear pain. At the doctor's office, the nurse finds that Audrey's ears are so full of wax that she is unable to see inside. Audrey, with her throbbing ear pain, is understandably terrified of the procedure the nurse does to help break up her wax and remove it. Bradley promises Audrey a treat and brags to everyone around about her bravery. Seeing Bradley with Audrey, I am struck by what a caring father he is. He quizzes her using her favorite book about unicorns. "What color is that one? And how many of them are purple?" Stroking her hair, he calls Rhonda so that Audrey can talk to her on the phone to help calm her.

Bradley confesses to me that he hates always being the parent who is around during painful times, because it makes him the bad guy, while Rhonda is seen as the fun parent. However, seeing Audrey cling to him and squeal when he tickles her and promises her a pink purse after the appointment ("She is so spoiled; you have no idea"), I am not convinced she views him as the bad cop. They arm-wrestle and Audrey wins. Throughout the appointment, he never skips a beat or misses an opportunity for a teaching moment with Audrey. Audrey points at the ear scope and says, "I hate that. I am so scared of it." Bradley tells her not to be afraid of doctors or their tools, because they are there to help us get better.

Coming from a huge family is a source of support and joy for Bradley. He has so many people who are there for him, who are available to help, and who are constantly worrying about him. Watching football and basketball games with his loved ones is a major way that he relaxes and finds a way to feel normal. At the same time, with his new position as a vulnerable, suffering member of the family, he feels alienated and lonely amidst such a large group. Even more painful than alienation to Bradley is feeling like a burden to his loved ones. "The one thing about being sick is you never have the right people to talk to. People are dealing with God knows how many problems. It's hard to add to that. I never want to tell anyone anything about my illness except to say when I'm in the hospital."

It doesn't appear that he has gotten used to feeling like a burden, but he has gotten good at hiding his symptoms, so as to appear as normal as possible. Bradley's people-pleasing personality occasionally creates a barrier between his primary care doctor, Dr. Castle, and him. A doctor-patient relationship rides on understanding and honesty. At times, Bradley nods enthusiastically and tells Dr. Castle that he understands a treatment plan, only to respond with confusion when Dr. Castle checks up on it with him a week later. When Bradley has brought up a problem or question to me, I often say, "Have you talked to Dr. Castle about that?" to which he replies, "No, I don't want to bother him with that." This behavior seems reasonable for anyone who becomes a chronic care patient, and has to suddenly grapple with new needs and problems. Dr. Castle has taken to writing down the issues and plans he goes over in appointments, and giving this outline to Bradley, which seems like a useful way to improve understanding and communication.

With many chronic conditions (as opposed to acute incidents) over time, the "Wow" factor wears off, the pity lessens, and the condition becomes a part of who the person is. Chronic illnesses may come crashing in, but they progress to remain a constant part of the lives of patients and their loved ones. People must normalize these continual conditions. At the same time, it can be hard for those who are sick to deal with something they despise becoming part of what defines them. For Bradley, the only thing he can have some control over is how others perceive his illness. Bradley works hard to make it seem like it's not a big deal—like lupus is not a defining trait of his. He doesn't want his family to visit him in the hospital, to paint their impression of him as a man in a hospital gown hooked up to an IV.

As much as Bradley tries to avoid "bothering" others with his symptoms, chronic illness does extend to impact all with whom an individual has contact. In the end, with chronically ill patients and their loved ones, a balance is reached, where the disease is accepted as part of their lives and a sense of normalcy and routine is returned. For this to happen, a great deal of effort needs to be made to redefine the roles of everyone involved. Bradley laments that chronic illness is "like a job. I wish I were getting paid." Except most regular jobs end each day and we go home. Chronic-care patients work overtime, can never quit, and cannot change their "employment" or choose a different boss. With lupus as Bradley's "cruel boss," his capabilities and interactions are restricted; and his time is shifted to take on new responsibilities in caring for himself. The roles and relationships that have defined his life must also change to accommodate the new "job" and its restrictions.

Bradley and his fiancé adjusted so that he took on more responsibility with the kids and at home, giving her an opportunity to pick up hours to better support them financially. They adapted and redefined this difficult circumstance into something positive that maintains some order and normalcy in their family. The family still watches sports together, and Bradley and Rhonda take advantage of his parents to drop the kids off and have date nights. On one such "date weekend," Bradley had an intense flare, but he and Rhonda were still able to appreciate the time alone, relaxing together—the epitome of adjusted expectations and skewed definitions of normalcy.

Rhonda is a huge source of support for Bradley. He says she has been there for him "from day one," helping him through the tears and pain and nausea. He respects and appreciates her sympathy, because of her own experiences as a patient. She was in a horrific car accident years ago, which left her in a month-long coma and with both femurs broken. Although Bradley finds great comfort in the fact that she understands being a patient, to an outsider, like me, there is a salient divide between her and his experiences with the healthcare system—hers being due to an acute trauma and his to a long-term chronic condition.

Rhonda is his ally and support, but Bradley makes it clear that he keeps a lot bottled up. Bradley often comments that Rhonda has been through much worse than him with her accident, and that his condition also puts her through a lot of pain, so he doesn't think it's fair to complain. "I am not a shy person, but I tend to hold my pain and feelings deep inside," he says. Because he keeps his feelings inside, I would argue that Bradley gets most of his support from himself. His self-therapy and his sense of humor combine with his intense desire to get better as a cocktail of strength and optimism, to overcome the terrifying pain he suffers. However, it is Bradley's family that kept him going on the days when he wondered what it would be like if he were gone. Although his coping strategies come from within, the strength and inspiration for the battle comes from his family.

Uncertainty often goes hand-in-hand with chronic conditions. An unpredictable progression is paired with erratic or ambiguous symptoms, to make planning for the future impossible. With chronic conditions, uncertainty about symptomatology spreads to uncertainty about treatment and uncertainty about one's relationships. In a condition like lupus, with periods of remission followed by exacerbation, making plans for the future is impossible. A glimpse into a year in Bradley's life, with exposure to his ups and downs, has shown me that, sometimes, the inability to plan for the future is more disabling than the physical consequences of the condition itself. When Bradley seems fine, when things are looking up, when he is in remission and capable, it is tempting to say that things are not so bad for him. However, it is the roller-coaster nature of lupus that makes the "good" times bittersweet. Even though he feels relatively well during remissions, he can never know how long they will last, thus crippling Bradley of the ability to set goals and begin projects or new tasks. He is never "normal" or fully capable, even when he is not technically experiencing a flare.

Recently, Bradley's blood tests came back showing that his disease is less active. He is in remission! He stopped the steroids he took for four years. While job-hunting, he is taking online classes to finish up an associate degree in psychology and community work. Mentally, he feels that he could go back to his old job, but physically he does not think he could handle it anymore. So he is looking elsewhere. Rhonda just got a new job as a graphic designer, her first job in her degree-field. Until now, she has worked at a scholastic program with teenage girls, helping them with their college applications and SATs. Bradley is excited for her to finally have her dream job, and for her to have a better paying one. His diabetes is under control, and he has not had a lupus flare-up in months. After a frustrating delay, he is once again starting up the pre-surgery steps he needs to take for his weight-loss surgery. He and his physicians are considering a band that wraps around the stomach and makes it seem smaller, instead of the stomach bypass, because it often involves fewer complications. This is another decision that reflects intense consideration and debate between care-team members.

Bradley and I have a very casual and friendly relationship, and Dr. Castle often reminds me to cherish this opportunity to get to know a patient with so few boundaries and constraints. It is, perhaps, my last chance for a patient to open up to me with no qualms or stilted communication from a pre-conceived power differential or notions of appropriate behavior. One reason I have an opportunity to get to know Bradley on a more personal level than I ever will get to know a patient when I practice as a physician is inherent in my project goal—to get to know him rather than to treat him. The lack of professional boundaries and lack of a precedent lets us create our relationship to be whatever we want.

As a physician, I recognize that I won't have this freedom, that I will be bound by preconceived notions, power differentials, and, appropriately, a focus on treating people rather than hanging out with them. Everyone has his or her own preset view of the doctor-patient relationship. Stereotypes exist for doctors, which force patients to act a certain way that is less real than in their encounters with friends. The power differential also creates a friction that forces doctors and patients out of their element. I am nervous about my future as a physician, when it will not be appropriate (not to mention, I won't have the time) to establish these types of friendships with my patients. If I don't get to know my patients this deeply, how will I understand them and be able to treat them? It seems difficult enough to treat as complex a patient as Bradley, even with a good understanding of his background.

This being said, some of these inevitable boundaries and accepted behaviors are necessary and good. As grateful as I am for Bradley's openness with me now, I can imagine that, as a physician, I probably won't want my patient to text me, "My daughter has an earache," at 10 p.m. on a Monday. This has been the beauty of my experience. I know that I will never again have the opportunity to truly gain a patient's thorough and raw perspective like this. I feel I have learned more from Bradley than from any class or experience in my first year. I hope the memory of Bradley's experience is with me for each test I order and every prescription I write, reminding me of the consequences of my actions on my patients as they work their way towards their definition of health. Before labeling a patient as "non-compliant," I hope I remember the scented bags Bradley carried everywhere he went. Bradley has taught me just how difficult compliance can be. For procedures that I might consider minor, I hope I remember Bradley's fear of the needle for checking his blood glucose. For him, an excruciatingly painful lupus flare is less scary than a needle stick. Bradley has been a daily reminder of just how different each person's psychological and physical thresholds can be.

Orders and prescriptions that look simple on paper have a new meaning, now that I have spent some time with Bradley. Most importantly, I have been reminded that a patient's life stretches outside of the exam room. Bradley is a tangible reminder that, when healthcare providers are away, patients continue struggling to achieve the elusive health that it is our job to augment. Bradley is not his illness. He is a Celtics fan, an avid reader, a family man. He loves psychology and children. Hilarious and calm, he is too proud to share his pains with those around him. He is struggling financially, psychologically, and physically. Shaped by a life of working for others and giving up his own wants and needs, his past has informed his experience as a patient. Relevant to many of my future patients, he is a person for whom health is no longer a given. His life was violently uprooted, forcing him to start over, redefine himself, and reorient his goals, values, and behaviors.

Bradley has shown me that medical treatment can be as violent and challenging as the illness. Saying "no" to medicine sometimes is not a sign that a patient has given up. Sometimes, there is great courage in choosing to live rather than choosing to fight for survival. And sometimes, life with medicine is more painful and difficult than life without. While Bradley's story is a gruesome reminder of how ugly medicine can be, it is also an uplifting testament to the power of patient education within a strong patient-doctor relationship. Bradley and Dr. Castle have taught me that, in medicine, failure is not a simple concept. Again, a physician's role is to help an individual achieve his or her own understanding of health. In Bradley's case, the lack of a cure, the inability to find the optimal treatment, the misdiagnosis, do not have be defined as failures but, rather, as opportunities to redefine health for each patient, and care for the messy scars left by life and medicine.

Vesuvius

GRACE LEE

Sometimes, while I'm riding the bus or walking down the street, I find myself gazing at passerby and wondering who they are, where they're going, what's on their mind. What gets them out of bed in the morning? What worries them? What motivates them? Are they happy? In the public context, my imaginative people-watching is simply out of curiosity. But in the medical setting, knowledge of what makes patients tick, what is important to them, what challenges they face every day are useful not only in terms of connecting with the patients, but also for refining diagnoses and treatment plans. Having grown up with someone who has a chronic illness, I knew first-hand the pain and the joy that comes with coping with a disease every minute of every day. I vowed to never forget that my patients are people too, with families and friends that love them, and with hopes and dreams that span beyond being physically healthy.

As I sat in my mentor's office, the selection of this patient was making me nervous. What if the patient and I don't form a connection? What if I am emotionally overwhelmed by the patient's condition? Just as the questions started spinning, Dr. Davis looked up with a smile. "Maryann would be perfect," he said. According to Dr. Davis, she was "interesting" and I would like her. His confidence was heartening, and my worries began to ebb. He turned to me and said, with a mischievous smile, "Don't forget to ask her to introduce you to Vesuvius!"

Maryann and I arranged to meet for the first time at a Starbucks near the hospital. I was worried that I wouldn't be able to recognize her, and would have to stand awkwardly in a corner and half-smile at random people until we happened to find each other. My worry was unfounded; I knew who she was the second I stepped into the café.

Maryann was perched uncomfortably on a stool, as young, fashionable, 20-somethings swirled around her, laughing and sipping lattes. She appeared so tiny and frail, yet her eyes were bright as she gazed inquisitively around the room. Wisps of gray hair peeked out from under a black, wool cap emblazoned with the words "Midnight Run." Her gray "Run for Research" sweatshirt was unzipped, revealing a neon-orange "Love Your Liver Run" sweatshirt underneath. Jeans with the cuffs rolled up, thick wool socks, and old black sneakers rounded out the ensemble.

She jumped up with a smile to shake my hand, and soon we were on our way—me with a Starbucks holiday drink and Maryann with a vente cappuccino with extra foam. It was her first coffee in months; she held the cup against her face with both hands, smiling as the aroma wafted around her. As she profusely thanked me for buying her the coffee, we wandered over to the Children's Hospital lobby to sit down for a chat.

Maryann opened up surprisingly quickly, frankly talking about everything from her operations and hospital stays to the Red Sox and Celtics, from her battles with diseases to her passions for knitting and running marathons. The conversation meandered comfortably, only broken by a few awkward silences that were quickly filled. I was struck by her cheerfulness, the brightness with which she described situations that would have been other people's worst nightmare. For a tiny, 60-year old woman, she certainly had spunk and a quirky sense of humor. Since this was our first meeting, I knew she had her guard up, and I was probably not seeing her true personality, but I was intrigued.

From this first meeting and our subsequent meetings and conversations, I was able to piece together Maryann's story, or at least the parts of which I was privileged enough to catch a glimpse.

ACCEPTANCE

Maryann was a retired teacher. For over two decades, she worked with mentally disabled students at a city school, whom she patiently taught anything and everything, ranging from colors and numbers to fine motor skills and toilet training. Despite the emotional nature of her work, she enjoyed her time teaching, fondly recalling particularly rambunctious children and adventures with kids in wheelchairs during fire drills. She ultimately retired, allowing her to concentrate on her new love: running.

Anyone who has talked to Maryann for more than five minutes knows that she lives for running. Her eyes light up at the mere mention of a marathon, and nearly every article of clothing she has is branded with the name of a race. Running brings structure to her life; every morning, she wakes up before 4 a.m. for an early morning run and carefully planned workout session at her local gym. More than just dedication and discipline, she is driven by a passion for running that grows with every passing day.

It all began a decade ago. Maryann has always loved to exercise and, at the time, she would go to the pool for two hours every day, either before or after work. For those two hours, she would swim back and forth, back and forth, back and forth, and she was content with that. One day, a flyer appeared in the pool locker room, advertising the first "Monster Triathlon" to be held in Boston. Maryann looked at the flyer and told herself, "You know you want the t-shirt for this." With that, she joined a relay team and signed up to do the swimming leg of the triathlon.

The athletes would be swimming in Boston Harbor, which Maryann thought was "so cool," but they were told that if, for some reason, they could not use the harbor, the triathlon would become a run-bike-run race. Maryann's first thought was, "What?! I can't run!" Everything ended up working out and she swam in Boston Harbor, but she thought to herself that next time she wanted to run too. The next year, she went to the

Boston Marathon expo and bought running shoes, running socks, and a book with tips on how to train yourself to run long distances. Following the book's techniques, she began running and at one point realized, "I like this." She thrived on the feeling of running outdoors, feeling her legs churning as she flew down the sidewalk, and before she knew it, she was addicted.

Maryann immediately entered herself in all the local races. Unlike before, when she would only participate in walkathons, or when she would walk race routes in order to raise money for the sponsoring charities, she could not wait to run. The Road Runners club had set up a tent at most of these races, and she decided to apply to join them. The running community welcomed her with open arms. Many of Maryann's training partners ran marathons and encouraged her to participate as well. She eagerly rose to the challenge and ran her first marathon just one year after starting to run. Now an experienced runner, she has completed 15 marathons total, including nine Boston marathons, with her best time being 4 hours, 28 minutes, in Chicago.

From her morning runs, to her lifting, spinning, rowing, and boxing classes, running and working out has become Maryann's life. The reactions of her doctors to her active lifestyle range from bemusement to enthusiasm; it was quite amusing for me to observe their responses to her excited descriptions of training. Her primary-care physician carefully questioned her about the extent of her workouts.

"How far are you running?" he asked.

"My long run is six miles now."

"Oh, good, six miles. . . . How long total is the marathon?"

"Oh, the whole thing? Twenty-six miles."

"That's what I was afraid of," he said with a rueful smile. Looking at her with probing eyes, he pushed her to describe her training plan. Watching him converse with Maryann, I respected the way he supported her love of running, while also ensuring the protection of her health.

When asked about why she runs, Maryann immediately states that running makes her feel like she has some control over her body, both physically and mentally. She loves to tell herself, "I'm gonna take control of you, body. You're gonna run 26.2 miles." This need to be in command of her body drives Maryann every minute of every day, and as I unpacked her medical experiences, I began to see why.

Maryann first suspected that something might be wrong when she realized that she could not control her bowel movements. She remembers going to the bathroom before a relay race just to urinate, but ending up having diarrhea that seemed like it would never stop. Having fought off breast cancer, she was terrified that her symptoms were due to another form of cancer, and immediately contacted her primary care physician. Her doctor suggested withholding dairy products from her diet, which helped at first, but when the symptoms recurred, he made an appointment for her with a gastrointestinal specialist.

From Maryann's presentation, the specialist suspected some form of inflammatory bowel disease (IBD). She had an examination of her bowels (a colonoscopy), which showed the entire bowel was inflamed. This condition was labeled as extensive, ulcerative colitis (UC), which is severe, advanced inflammation, or colitis. Nevertheless, Maryann was immensely relieved when she was diagnosed with colitis because, as a breast cancer survivor, she had feared that the cancer had returned. She has no ideas as to what could have led to her colitis, and does not seem particularly concerned about pinpointing the cause. She read somewhere that Jewish people are more likely to develop ulcerative colitis but, though she is Jewish, no one in her family had any GI problems. To this day, not even the experts are sure what causes ulcerative colitis. Some have suggested that it is a type of immune disorder, while others have proposed that the colitis is due to an abnormal response to normal intestinal bacteria. Genetics appear to be related to people's risk of developing the disease, though it is still being investigated.

At the time of her diagnosis, Maryann already had the classic symptoms of colitis: frequent bowel movements, diarrhea with mucus, urgency, and incontinence. Unfortunately, the medical management of UC is far from perfect, and Maryann experienced that first hand. Maryann met with a general surgeon to discuss the surgical options for her disease. Most surgery for this condition involves the removal of some or all of the colon. Surgery not only cures the disease, it also reduces the risk of developing a cancer and decreases the need to take medications over the long-term, but it does drastically alter the patient's lifestyle and appearance. When the diarrhea continued despite increased medications, Maryann decided to undergo the operation. In the meantime, despite her medical issues, Maryann participated in the Boston Marathon. As if to reaffirm her decision to get the surgery, she was only able to run the first two miles; her diarrhea became so bad, she was forced to walk the remainder of the marathon, crossing the finish line over eight hours later. When looking back on that day, she often remarks, "It's funny to see a marathon after it's been cleaned up!"

The surgeon removed Maryann's colon and rectum, and created a new rectum, called a pouch, by using the small bowel with a temporary stoma. The stoma, or opening, is an outlet of the bowel on the abdomen, with a collection bag for stool. Once the pouch has healed, the stoma is closed and the patient can resume regular bowel movements. Maryann remembers waking up after the surgery and feeling great, like she could conquer the world. Looking down at her brand new stoma encased in an ostomy bag, she "didn't think it was that bad." She went home five days after surgery, with the promise of another procedure in a few months to close the stoma.

Maryann was delighted with the results of the surgery. She no longer had to worry about diarrhea spilling out of her "Big Bird" diapers, and she was no longer confined to her apartment after eating. She could eat peanut butter again! Figuring out how to manage the stoma bag—how to prevent the bag from leaking and what to do if and when it leaked—was a challenge, but a welcome dilemma given the alternative. A visiting nurse came by her apartment frequently after the surgery to teach her how to care for the stoma, and Maryann had regular appointments with a stoma nurse at the hospital. It was during a visit with the stoma nurse that her ileostomy "erupted" with stool, thus leading her to name the stoma (Maryann decided the ileostomy was female) "Vesuvius," or "Suvie" for short. (In contrast, according to Maryann, many patients name their ostomies after ex-boyfriends or girlfriends, because "shit goes through them.")

The most common complication of an ileostomy is skin irritation around the opening. Also, patients with ileostomies become dehydrated very easily, a particular concern for Maryann given her active lifestyle. Though not a complication, sometimes mucus is passed through the rectum. The surgeon had warned Maryann about the mucus, but she was still not prepared to wake up in the middle of the night with "black stuff" all over her bed, precipitating a frantic 3 a.m. phone call to the eminently patient surgeon.

Two months after the surgery, Maryann had the ileostomy closure, which went smoothly, and she returned home from the hospital five days later. However, almost immediately after she was discharged, Maryann began having bouts of abdominal pain, nausea, and vomiting. Though she felt terrible, she assumed that her symptoms were due to the healing process, and tried to grit her teeth and wait it out. But when the pain became worse and she developed a fever, she knew something was going on, and called for an ambulance to take her to the hospital. Maryann was taken to the emergency department, where they found an obstruction of the bowel. When she did not improve after a few days of rest, the surgeon decided to take Maryann back to the OR. There was obstruction or blockage of the bowel by scar tissue and a small perforation or leak. The surgeon released the blockage, closed the perforation, and created a new stoma.

When Maryann woke up, Vesuvius was back. Disheartened, she took longer to recover, eventually being discharged 10 days after she had been rushed to the hospital in an ambulance. Slowly, reluctantly, she returned to her life of working out and caring for her stoma. It was at that point, two months after her bowel obstruction ordeal, that I met Maryann. From the start, her proactive, careful management of her stoma and the extent to which she had adapted to life with Vesuvius impressed me. Knowing that her lack of a colon put her at increased risk of dehydration, particularly given her daily workouts, she always maintained a healthy stock of Gatorade. She never left her apartment without an extra ostomy bag, toilet paper, an extra pair of pants, and an adult diaper. Her conversations with her stoma nurse revealed her thorough knowledge of the world of ostomies: They bantered about the various ostomy bag suppliers, the pros and cons of different types of bags, and tricks for preventing leakage. Maryann carefully examined her stoma every day, checking her skin for signs of irritation and asking Vesuvius how she was doing.

By all appearances, Maryann seemed lighthearted and cheerful, taking her ileostomy in stride, and joking that she could "scare teenage boys" with it. But it was the rare moments in between her upbeat comments when she fell silent, revealing her internal struggle. The decision of whether or not to close her stoma again weighed on her mind. Taking care of the bag was a hassle, but one she was prepared to deal with for the rest of her life, if necessary. Though she longed to be free of the bag, the idea of undergoing the ileostomy closure and having it fail a second time terrified her. She never wanted to go through that ordeal again. Yet the task of maintaining the ostomy bag, day in and day out, began taking a toll, and her spirit began to wear thin. Ultimately, she decided to try one more time, and scheduled her stoma closure with the surgeon for a week after the Boston Marathon.

Two months before the marathon, Maryann invited me over to her apartment. I ventured across town on a chilly, rainy day in February. Maryann lives alone on the third floor of a cute little house, wedged between two other cute little houses, in an old but well-maintained suburb of Boston. When she opened the door for me at the bottom of the stairs, I was struck again by just how tiny she was. She walked quickly up the steep stairs, which were lit from above by a skylight, casting the staircase in a cold, white light.

We arrived on the third floor, kicked off our shoes, and entered her apartment. In her foyer, I was immediately struck by the colorful posters on the walls, the knick-knacks hanging from the door frames, and the running trophies piled on a table. I felt pulled in a million directions; I wanted to ask her about everything! But beneath my excitement and fascination, I felt a sense of discomfort. Something was off. I pushed the feeling out of my mind and walked into an adjoining room. Various pieces of artwork hung on the walls, but a large pastel dominated the room. Drawn on a dark background, red, brown, and grey tendrils undulated gracefully across the canvas, coming together to form an elegantly branching structure that could have been a tree. Maryann gave it half a glance and explained that a friend made it for her years ago. The other pieces of colorful artwork were items she had found at local crafts fairs.

She hovered in the doorway, seemingly impatient to move to the other side of the apartment.

Gazing around this large room, which looked like it could have been the master bedroom, I realized what was troubling me. Boxes were neatly stacked against the walls and in the center of the room. The windows were bare of curtains. The floor surrounding the boxes was empty. There was no furniture. Maryann apologized for the mess, explaining that bed bugs had invaded her apartment last year, and she hadn't had time to unpack again after the exterminators came through. She seemed a bit self-conscious, and I gave her a reassuring smile, though I worried about how she could be living in a place that felt so empty.

We walked through the foyer, which also had half-open boxes neatly pushed to the center of the room, and peeked into the bathroom. Maryann's a tiny lady, but looking into that minuscule room, I wondered if even she could maneuver in there. Small glimpses of tiled floor were barely visible under the boxes of ostomy bag supplies. Wafers of every size, used to connect the bag to the skin around her stoma, were piled on the floor, next to extra ostomy bags and adult diapers. "I'm ready for anything," she said proudly.

Adjacent to the tiny bathroom were the kitchen and her bedroom. Walking into the kitchen, I felt my entire body relax. Here was the clutter I was expecting, the cozy lived-in feeling that I was hoping to see. Marathon posters and runners' bibs were plastered all over the walls. Colorful wall hangings and light-switch covers depicting frolicking cats covered the cabinets. A quirky clock was frozen in time next to a wall calendar that was diligently covered in sticky notes detailing all of Maryann's training sessions, doctor's appointments, and occasional get-togethers with friends. Red and orange Gatorade bottles, which she was stockpiling in preparation for the Boston Marathon and recovery after her surgery, lined a wall.

Photos of her niece and nephew as young children and adults were gathered on a small table, above cookbooks that were clearly not seeing much use. A small radio broadcasting local sports talk buzzed merrily in the background. Though there were boxes piled in the center of the room, they were mostly unpacked, and there was no sharp divide between the island of boxes and the rest of the room.

On the door between the bedroom and the kitchen, Maryann had fashioned a rack of sorts, upon which to hang her numerous medals. Ribbons of all colors and medals of all shapes and sizes cheerfully clanked into each other, like a set of wind chimes, which Maryann gazed at in pride. "Oh, they're just finishing medals," she said modestly, though I saw at least two first-place awards.

Unlike the kitchen, Maryann's bedroom also seemed disconcertingly sparse, with her dresser on one side of the room and her bed—just a mattress and a pile of sheets and blankets—pushed into a corner of the floor. She walked right by the bed without a glance and picked up a small picture frame. "Want to see my cats?" she asked, with a bright smile. "Here's Thomas James, that's Thomasina Shermanetta, and that's Felix." She looked wistfully at the picture, her eyes lingering on her favorite, Thomasina, named after two Celtics players, who died of cancer. If the surgery goes well, she plans on getting another cat and finding a part-time job because "cats can be expensive."

We returned to the kitchen and settled down for a chat. Maryann immediately jumped up to make tea, heating up the water in an ancient-looking kettle and pouring the tea into large flowery mugs. After she updated me on her training (she had just started a boxing class and was tapering down her running in preparation for the marathon), I gently asked her about how she was feeling mentally. With hardly a pause, she said that she is usually able to joke about her condition, but certainly some days she "just wants to hide in bed." I nodded, hoping that she would continue. But she quickly moved on, saying that she is actually quite grateful, as some people develop ulcerative colitis much younger in life. And with that, the moment of vulnerability had passed.

I had been wondering for a while about whether Maryann was truly happy. She certainly wanted to make it seem like she was. But I had the nagging sensation that she was hiding her feelings of loneliness, helplessness. Whether her façade was conscious or not, I knew there was more to her than just strength and self-sufficiency. Despite my curiosity, I respected her clear desire to avoid dwelling on her negative emotions. Perhaps it was another aspect of her drive to control her body; she could master it in a physical sense, by making it run a marathon, and in a mental sense, by pushing out unwanted feelings.

Or, perhaps, I was over-thinking it. As Maryann showed me out of her apartment, I felt her relax, like the type of relief you feel after entertaining guests, when you close the door and your home is your own again. Her home was her kingdom; everything was in its proper place, optimized for her lifestyle and habits. Perhaps I was projecting my emotions on to her, assuming that she was feeling lonely and depressed, when she may have been exactly as content and independent as she appeared. I certainly hoped so. I was becoming very fond of Maryann, and did not want to picture her sitting alone with just her thoughts in her cold apartment.

Marathon Monday dawned bright and clear. I sat in lecture, twitching, staring at the clock, counting down the time until I could escape into the warm sunshine and see Maryann run. Ten o'clock, the start of the race, came and went as I absent-mindedly took notes. Maryann had registered my cell phone number with the marathon organizers, enabling me to receive text messages when she passed 10 km, 25 km, 30 km, and the finish line. My phone buzzed and my heart leaped at 11:45am;

Maryann had just passed the 10 km mark. I pictured her tiny figure running amidst a crowd of other marathoners, and longed to join the cheering onlookers. Class finally ended at 12:30 p.m. and I was out the door by 12:31 p.m. My friends and I made our way to Kenmore Square, where the marathon festivities were in full swing. The marathon path was packed with runners, cheered from all sides by college students, families, and young adults decked out in Red Sox gear. Onlookers crowded the windows and roof-decks of nearby buildings, barbecues were churning out burgers and hot dogs, and music was blasting from all directions. The air felt electric with excitement, pride, energy.

I grabbed an empty spot on the fence as my phone buzzed again; Maryann had just passed 25 km. She was more than halfway done! I knew she still had a while to go before she reached me, as I was standing at the 25-mile mark, but I could not help eagerly scanning the crowd for her small figure, her wispy gray hair. Though this was not the first time I had been to the Boston Marathon, I was struck anew by the incredible variety of runners. Twenty-somethings in the best shape of their lives ran alongside lean and wiry middle-aged men and women. A group of soldiers in army fatigues and carrying huge packs marched along the side of the path, their heads held high, smiling at the cheers of "USA! USA!" People wearing Children's Hospital jerseys sprinted by a man in a ballet tutu, who, in turn, passed a man in a cowboy hat. A man with a prosthetic leg ran by, flanked by two guides wearing bright, yellow shirts, as my friends and I gazed in amazement.

An hour of cheering and high-fiving passed in the blink of an eye. My phone beeped; Maryann had passed 30 km. Now there would be no more text messages until she reached the finish line. I bounced on the balls of my feet, excited to see her in all of her running glory. Another hour passed and the crowd of runners and onlookers slowly thinned. Most of the runners were charity runners, wearing t-shirts and jerseys supporting their various causes. More and more bandit runners—people who did not officially register to run the race, but jumped the fence somewhere along the route—appeared, sprinting bibless by police officers who just shook their heads and let them pass. A blind runner cruised by, also flanked by guides in bright yellow, one of whom was carrying a short rope that the blind man held for guidance. Many runners were accompanied by friends and family who had hopped the fence, sprinting alongside their loved ones in flip-flops and jeans, waving their arms to encourage onlookers to cheer. Yet still there was no Maryann.

Another hour came and went. The temperature began to drop, and the sky became overcast. I maintained my watchful position by the fence, hoping to see Maryann with each passing minute. Worry began to creep into my mind. What if something happened? What if Vesuvius was acting up? What if she had to stop running for some reason? What if she fainted from dehydration? It didn't help that my recent exam in physiology class focused on a marathon runner who had seizures due to low sodium levels. I tried to push aside my fears, telling myself that with all of the police officers and EMTs posted along the route, she would be fine. But I grew quieter, hardly cheering as I began scanning the few remaining runners for Maryann's face.

I paced along the fence, mostly to stay warm, but never taking my eyes off of the runners. I ran into several friends from college who delightedly began asking me about medical school, and I chatted with them while still trying to look for Maryann. Not wanting to appear rude, I grudgingly turned my focus to the conversation. I don't know what made me turn, but a few minutes later, I whipped around just in time to see a runner in a bright orange baseball hat running away from me. It had to be Maryann—the wispy gray hair, the slight figure, the determination that seemed to lift her up with each stride. I couldn't make out what was written on her legs and back, but I cheered with all of my strength. Pride warmed me to my core, and I knew I had just witnessed one of the most inspirational moments of my life.

My friends and I strolled toward the Westin hotel in Copley Square, where Maryann said I could find her after the race. My phone beeped one final time; Maryann had just finished her ninth Boston marathon in 5 hours and 41 minutes, averaging 13 minutes a mile. Not bad for a 60-year-old woman who weighs less than 100 lbs, is missing a colon, and has a stoma named Vesuvius.

I found Maryann triumphantly eating a peanut butter and jelly bagel, wrapped in the unmistakable foil poncho that marked the champions of Marathon Monday, still with the bright-orange Red Sox cap jammed on her head. The blue and yellow finisher's medal hung proudly around her neck. She chewed happily on her bagel, commenting that it was the first real food that she'd eaten all day. I congratulated her on her time, but she brushed it off, saying that she was hoping to get under 5 hours. Maybe next year, she said with a smile.

As she got up to go to one of the hotel rooms to shower, I noticed the writing on her legs. "Go Red Sox!" read her left calf, and "Go C's and B's" was scrawled on her right calf. "C's and B's?" I asked. "Celtics and Bruins," she replied, as though it was obvious. Her name was on the front of her shirt, and the names of her sponsors were on the back, along with "Vesuvius" written in large black letters. Seeing her thin legs poking out from under the foil, I was struck again by the knowledge that this tiny woman had run more in one day than most people run in a month.

I walked her to the elevator, still smiling and feeling like I would burst with pride. Maryann didn't seem fazed at all by her accomplishment. "Well, I guess I'd better do an easier workout tomorrow," she commented. "I need to make sure I'm ready for the surgery next week."

The day of Maryann's surgery arrived a short week later. As I woke up, brushed my teeth, and threw on scrubs, the enormity of the moment did not dawn on me; it felt like any other day. I ran to the hospital and met Maryann and her friend Rosie in the family waiting area. Rosie, an ultramarathoner, always drives Maryann to the hospital on the mornings of her surgeries, and waits until she has word that the operation went well. Even as I sat there, chatting with them about running and gossiping about people in the marathon community, it felt like any other day. Watching Maryann nervously knitting, I tried to make myself feel something, empathize with her fears. But the sense of normalcy would not go away.

Sooner than I expected, we were summoned to pre-op. As we walked through the doors, Maryann said that it was "so nice to walk in here, and not be on a stretcher." While Rosie and I hovered in the area outside of her bed, trying not to obstruct the carefully-designed flow of the room, Maryann put on a hospital gown. The vulnerability was back: her tiny figure wrapped in the huge gown, her wispy hair pulled back into a thin braid that she kept winding around her finger, and her bright eyes moving from person to person in excitement tinged with nervousness.

Whenever anyone approached her, Maryann blurted out her name and birth date unprompted, eliciting smiles and "you know the drill" comments. Rosie and I kept chatting with her about marathons, as nurses and anesthesiologists swirled around us. The surgeon, jovially humming, and the resident appeared, checking on Maryann before she was taken to the OR. Amidst the hustle and bustle, Maryann was perched on the bed hiding her nervousness behind a brave face. I could sense her worry, but I still could not make myself feel the gravity of the moment.

A short while later, right on schedule, Maryann was wheeled to the OR. She was quickly lifted onto the operating table, where she was covered with blankets and told to put her head on the "life-saver" pillow. Through the whole process, Maryann was very quiet. I hovered nearby, adjusting her blankets, helping where I could, but otherwise staying out of the way. The anesthesiologist administered the sedative and, within seconds, Maryann fell asleep. The tension seemed to flow out of her face; her eyes relaxed, the surrounding wrinkles becoming more prominent as her eyelids closed. Her mouth fell slack, slightly open, a glimmer of a smile visible through the facemask. I was mesmerized by the calmness and contentment that radiated from her face. The anesthesiologist interrupted my brief reverie, whisking off the facemask, taping Maryann's eyelids to protect her eyes during surgery, and placing a breathing tube.

The pace of the room quickened as the surgeon walked in. Maryann's abdomen was exposed and her ileostomy bag removed, revealing Vesuvius, a nubbin of wrinkly pink bowel peeking out from a hole in her abdominal wall. The surgical resident sutured the opening in the ileostomy closed, and the circulating nurse prepped the skin of her abdomen with antiseptic. Everyone commented on Maryann's tiny physique; she looked almost skeletal on the operating table, with her pelvis jutting out on either side of her concave abdomen. Then everyone scrubbed, they placed the drapes, the resident asked for a scalpel, and I braced myself for the incision. I winced as the resident carefully cut an incision around the stoma. But as the procedure continued, my qualms faded quickly. With the drapes up and Maryann's face covered, this felt almost like every other time I had shadowed in the operating room. The operation proceeded smoothly, with the surgeon cheerfully instructing the resident throughout.

As the anesthesiologist woke Maryann, I saw her arms move at first, and then her eyes open. I will never forget the look on her face as she awoke—a mixture of confusion, alarm, fear. Her eyes were huge and luminous and fixed on me; in my surprise, I wondered if she recognized me. I smiled and murmured that the procedure had gone well, but her eyes never faltered, never lost their look of panic. I looked at her, she looked at me; she did not say anything and I didn't know what to say. In that moment, the enormity of the event sank in. Maryann, my first patient, my friend, had just been opened up, her insides cut, poked, and prodded, and sewed up. Now she was waking up, terrified that something had gone wrong and that she was worse off than before. I may have known that it was just a minor procedure, but to Maryann it was something that could change her life, for the better or for the worse.

Maryann was soon moved to the recovery room, where I continued to reassure her. She began murmuring that she wanted to vomit, and though the nurse-anesthetist started her on some anti-nausea medications, the nausea and pain grew worse. She grimaced, shifted in the bed, and began to shiver and gag. I piled on more blankets and held a tray under her chin, feeling so helpless, so incapable of making her pain go away. Every few minutes she would open her eyes and look at me; I smiled in a way that I hoped was comforting, and told her that the medication should kick in soon. Finally, after what felt like an eternity, she started to look more comfortable. I quietly left so that Maryann could rest, telling her that I would come visit her again later that day.

When I returned to the hospital that night, Maryann looked tired but comfortable, nestled amidst a pile of blankets and pillows. She said that a bit of gas pain remained, and the nausea was mostly gone. It was incredibly comforting to see her so relaxed, already looking forward to eating normal food and walking around.

As I walked back to my dorm from the hospital, I reflected on the day, from the mundane morning, to Maryann's shocking fear and pain upon waking up, to her quiet recovery. Up until that point, I had only seen surgeries from the perspective of the surgeon—coming in to the OR after the patient was already under anesthesia, and leaving before the patient woke up. Spending the day with Maryann, I now appreciated the fear of undergoing an operation, no matter how trivial. I realized that, despite the hustle and bustle of pre-op and the presence of friends, patients often feel alone with their thoughts and their worries, a small cog in the fast-paced workings of the hospital. I hope to hold on to these thoughts, to never forget the look in Maryann's blue eyes as she awoke, as I proceed through the years of medical training.

It Is What It Is

ADA AMOBI

The first time I met Mike was at a rehabilitation center. It was late in the evening and the entire building was quiet. As I walked down the halls, I caught glimpses of the patients in some of the rooms with the doors open; most of them were in bed quietly watching television or eating dinner. As I came closer to Mike's room I was a little nervous. I had never met anyone with muscular dystrophy and did not know what to expect. I wanted to make a good first impression.

What immediately struck me when I stepped into his room was the plethora of tubes and contraptions that he was connected to. It was striking how the very things that were helping to keep him alive also appeared to be great nuisances. He had just finished dinner and was sitting in his chair. He wanted to go to the solarium down the hall to talk. It probably took about four minutes for his mother to disconnect him from some of his machines and reconnect him to a portable ventilator but it felt twice as long.

It appeared that Mike was not happy that he needed his mother's help. "No, I do not need that right now" he snapped when his mother tried to get him to wear a sensor to keep track of his oxygen levels. Mike's mom was a nurse and had the medical skills necessary to take care of him. In the months to come I would learn more about the complexities of the relationship between Mike and his parents. When he was settled in the solarium we started to talk about his journey from diagnosis to his stay in the rehabilitation center.

Mike did not really notice that he had a problem until he was 13 years old. Before then he only knew that he couldn't keep up with his peers. "I was about 9 years old in gym class and had to do 10 hurdles. I realized immediately that there was no way I was going to jump over the hurdle. I just knew that all of the kids were physically superior. I couldn't even come close."

He had another turning point when he was about 24 years old. He was driving and couldn't adequately control the car with his hands, lost control and ended up on someone's lawn. "It was one of those situations when you go, 'You know what? I should have done better.' You sit back and you think about that and you go, 'Okay, I could have hurt someone. I can't do this anymore'." Mike soon stopped driving altogether because of the growing difficulty with his reflexes. He was so shaken by that incident and the prospect of possibly hurting someone that he couldn't bring himself to drive again.

Mike did not start using a wheelchair until he found it more difficult to walk long distances. Whenever he went to large arenas for concerts or sports he would use a wheelchair. "I kept using it more and more until I broke my leg," Mike recalled. Fracturing his leg was the turning point; the day of the fracture would be the last day he spent outside of a wheelchair.

"It was really stupid," he recalled; he broke his leg as he was getting off of a couch. At that time, he routinely needed help rising up from couches. His father who would normally have helped him up was turned away and Mike attempted to get up on his own, tripped over his foot, and fell to the ground. He heard the crack and waited for the pain to subside but it remained excruciatingly painful. When I asked him about how that experience affected him emotionally, he said: "I cried for like three minutes and then I said to myself: 'It is what it is . . . there is nothing I can do about it'." After the six weeks of immobility due to his broken leg, Mike's muscles were no longer strong enough to walk. "I always knew it would happen," he said.

Mike's parents accepted their son's diagnosis with equanimity: "It was going to be what it was going to be," his father said, "It made no sense to be worried and it made no sense to be hopeful." His parents understood that each case of facio-scapulohumeral (FSHD) Muscular Dystrophy was so completely different that there was no way to predict how the disease would affect Mike. This genetic disorder results in progressive muscle weakness and atrophy. "We were going to wait and see," his dad explained. This attitude was instrumental in helping his family deal with the uncertain diagnosis. Mike's parents learned as much as they could from reading about the disease, as well as from the New England FSHD Society. Mike's mother was especially poised to be a good advocate for Mike because of her medical background and subsequent ease within the clinical environment.

I asked Mike's dad, Rick, what was the most challenging aspect of being a parent of someone with FSH Muscular Dystrophy. I expected him to talk about some of the stresses that it put on his family, either logistically or financially, or perhaps to talk about the difficulty in reconciling dreams and aspirations for Mike with the limitations that Mike's disorder has placed on him. Yet, for Rick, the biggest challenge was to let go of the parent role and to let Mike make his own decisions. Although Rick understood more than anyone that Mike was completely capable of making his own choices, it was still sometimes hard for Rick to refrain from imposing his will on Mike. "The most challenging thing has been to act in such a way to make sure Mike has the greatest opportunity to make his own decisions. As a parent you always want to jump in and it's not appropriate for us to do that. I'm still his father and will provide my opinion but, ultimately, there's more of a respectful relationship."

This relationship proved to be a great source of support for Mike especially when he was in the process of deciding whether or not to get a tracheostomy. The decision to get a tracheostomy or permanent breathing tube in the neck means being dependent on a breathing machine or ventilator to some extent. It means having to change the way you do everyday things like shave and eat. There are many reasons why a tracheostomy is used such as to bypass an obstruction in the airway, clean and remove mucus from the airway, and to deliver oxygen to the lungs easily and safely. In Mike's case, his Muscular Dystrophy paralyzed and weakened his chest wall. In addition, his neuromuscular disease made it hard for him to clear secretions and led to low oxygen levels. It became clear during a hospital stay for pneumonia, that he would need help to breathe, and the ventilator was his best bet.

Although a tracheostomy has benefits for patients and makes it easier for the medical team to provide breathing support, it comes with a lot of complications. Because the opening for the tracheostomy tube is essentially an open cut, there is a risk of infection. Scar tissue from the surgery can damage the windpipe. The tube can be blocked by pressure in the airway walls, blood clots or mucus and must be periodically suctioned to stay clean. Furthermore, there is a risk of damage to the esophagus and to the nerve that moves the vocal cords, thus, patients with tracheostomies may develop long-term difficulty swallowing or talking.

"Getting better faster was my main concern," Mike explained. While he was not happy with the short-term implications of using a tracheostomy, such as the dependence on a machine, he was thinking forward to the future, and believed that, in the long-term, the tracheostomy would help him get out of the hospital faster. When asked how he knew it was the decision for him, Mike replied, "It's a feeling in your gut, you just sort of know." He was worried about possible infections, and was not happy about having to be hooked up to a machine all day, but, after weighing the pros and cons, he realized that the tracheostomy made the most sense for him.

As with every other medical hurdle that Mike has experienced, his family was right there by his side. Mike's mom was fiercely protective and Rick, recalled that during that time in the hospital, she would require anyone who entered the room to explain who they were and why they were there. His parents always made sure that the doctors paid attention to Mike's wishes and explained the reasons behind their treatment plans. According to Rick, "Mostly, it's the physicians who fail to recognize that Mike has choices. *They often cross the line from being advisors to being advocates.*" Mike's parents were vigilant in making sure that doctors considered what was important to Mike.

The first time I met Mike he still had his tracheostomy in place and seemed to have grown accustomed to it. However he was anxious to get off of the ventilator as soon as he possibly could. The time Mike spent at the rehabilitation center was challenging for him. There, he was pushed to work hard. "It was like weight training," Mike explained; "every day you would do a period of time off the tracheostomy, and the next day you would do 5 percent more, and that was the program." By the time he was discharged from the rehabilitation center he was able to get up to 9-10 hours without using the trach, but he didn't stop there. "When I got home I was like: 'if I can do 10 hours I can do 12'." Mike pushed himself harder and harder to go longer and longer without the trach; he believes that the process of getting weaned off of a tracheostomy is 95% mental.

He was eventually able to get to the point where he was only using the tracheostomy at night. Although he was happy that he no longer had to be attached to the ventilator, there were still certain aspects of the tracheostomy opening in his neck that bothered him. "It's like a paper cut," he explained; "You nick it and then it gets better in a few minutes." The paper cuts he was referring to were the little nuisances that came along with having a tracheostomy stoma. Mike had to be careful when he was shaving to properly cover the wound and to keep hair from getting in. When he went out in the cold months he had to take extra measures to cover up his neck with multiple scarves. Taking a shower was also very difficult because he had to keep the wound dry. Each morning when Mike does all of the daily rituals that most of us take for granted, he is reminded that he is in fact different and that as much as he has tried to live a "normal" life he has not fully been able to achieve the normalcy he desires.

As his respiratory capacity steadily declined, one of the hardest things that Mike had to deal with was the fear and anxiety associated with his prognosis. Doctors and respiratory specialists constantly warned Mike that without a tracheostomy he could be facing dire consequences. One doctor who chose not to mince words said simply: "You could die." Indeed, because of the weakness of his respiratory muscles Mike could possible die in his sleep due to lack of proper ventilation.

It is hard to imagine what it must be like to face one's mortality in such a way. Sadness, anger, fear and anxiety are all emotions that I imagine I would feel if I was in the same situation. For Mike, his anxiety was a very strong and sometimes incapacitating emotion that gave him a lot of distress. Fortunately, Mike sought help from a pediatric palliative care specialist, Dr. Bloch, who also specialized in teaching techniques such as breathing, visualizations and other mental exercises. Dr. Bloch advised Mike to either take his mind to another time and place in which he felt comfort and serenity.

The method of going to a different place mentally is self-hypnosis. Through self-hypnosis, patients utilize scenes and mental images to help their anxiety subside. A health practitioner or hypnotist can give the patient examples of images to use, or the patient can provide his or his own direction. An example of a mental image that can be used for self-hypnosis is that of a calming pool. Dr. Bloch stressed the importance of letting Mike come up with his own images. She wanted to empower him to conquer his anxiety on his own terms. She also was careful to avoid mentioning muscle and breathing techniques that are commonly used in self-hypnosis since these would not be helpful to Mike considering his physical condition. "The more sensual, the more therapeutic," Dr. Bloch explained. It is important that when Mike goes to his mental refuge that he tries to imagine how it felt, smelled, and tasted to be there. Being able to manage his anxiety was an important step in helping Mike make sound medical decisions and have a better quality of life.

In my conversations with Mike he recounted some of his experiences with being viewed as "other" by people that he encountered. *"Some people look at you not like it's the legs—like it's your head; they talk down to you as if there's something wrong with you. Not everyone's a brain surgeon,"* he rationalized. He understood that some of the negative reactions that he had experienced stemmed from ignorance and not from maliciousness. Mike also found that some people, would not treat him as if he was mentally handicapped but instead would be compelled to share the personal stories with him, especially stories of misfortune. *"I could tell you stories of people who are kind of forward; they just unconsciously just come up and start telling me their life story . . . you get another segment of people that feel the need to tell you what's wrong with them so that they're trying to commiserate."* While Mike's wheelchair and ventilator equipment enable him to do many things, they can also be a great source of social isolation and can invite unwanted interactions. Mike fortunately views the unwanted interactions and comments with great equanimity and does not let the prospect of negative interactions keep him from being sociable.

It is impossible to fully understand what it means to live with FSH muscular dystrophy. There is a limit to how much someone without the disorder can understand; however, my many conversations with Mike really helped give me good insight into his world and an appreciation of what it means to have the disease.

ACCEPTANCE

One of the hardest and yet the best parts of practicing medicine is finding a way to connect with people who are completely different from you. Mike and I were different in many ways: our cultural and religious background, the types of towns we grew up in, and even the kind of music we liked. One of the most difficult differences in our lives to reconcile was the disparity between the things that we are each able to do, see and experience. Whenever Mike would ask me what was new in school I would find myself hesitating to talk about things that I knew he would never be able to do because of his ambulatory and respiratory restrictions. I would start telling him about a dance performance I was in or an event I took part in for the school's society Olympics and then find my excitement about recounting the story wane as I became acutely aware that the things I so vividly described were activities that he most likely could never do. I would find myself minimizing how enjoyable something was or quickly trying to change the subject. I realize now that while it is good to be sensitive to Mike's situation in life, I was wrong to think that by telling him about certain things I was somehow highlighting the fact that he was confined to a wheelchair. He would be aware of that regardless of what experiences I chose to share.

Although we were different in many ways, it was surprisingly easy to identify with Mike when he recounted certain feelings and experiences. For example, he once recounted a time when he was in a rehabilitation center and despite ringing the call bell numerous times no responded. He talked about how frustrated he was and how despite his frustration, he didn't want to complain because he was afraid that the staff would consciously or unconsciously retaliate as they continued his care in the future. While I have never had the experience of having hospital employees not respond to my call bell, and indeed, I have never even been hospitalized as an in-patient, I still was able to relate to the feelings of anger, frustration and fear that he experienced during that moment. There were many other instances like this when I found myself completely relating to Mike's feelings even though I couldn't exactly relate to his experiences.

Despite all I was able to learn this year, there are still many questions left unanswered and things I would have liked to see. For instance, since Mike lived far away in New Hampshire and I have no car, I wasn't able to go to his home and see him in his own natural surroundings. Although I wanted to learn more about his relationship with his mother and how she was able to balance the role of mother and medical professional, I wasn't able to speak with her because she declined an interview. Nevertheless, I was able to get a multifaceted view of Mike's story because I met and talked with several people in Mike's life that had completely different perspectives but all shared the same final goal of supporting Mike's health and wellbeing. Given privacy issues, I chose not to pass on the messages I received from one party to another but it was clear that if everyone could talk to each other and learn from one another, Mike's quality of care would be even better than it is.

One of the biggest lessons I learned about giving patients good quality care as a physician had to do with appreciating the gravity of medical decisions from the patient's perspective. As medical professionals (and medical professionals in training), it is easy to view invasive medical procedures as everyday occurrences. For a respiratory therapist or an ICU doctor a tracheostomy is a commonplace device, but for a patient getting a tracheostomy, it is a scary and invasive procedure. My conversations with Mike have taught me to strive to put myself in the patient's shoes when discussing treatment options in the future, to be sensitive to my patients' concerns and fears, and not treat medical decisions flippantly.

During the months I spent talking with Mike and with other people involved in his life and care, I constantly battled a feeling of voyeurism. At times I was afraid to encourage Mike to share about some difficult topics, such as when he became confined to a wheelchair, because I felt as though I was only taking from him and had nothing to give back. I know that if I was a member of his treatment team for example, I would feel better about delving into his past because the information I glean can be used to help him. In the context of this class however, I often felt as though I was learning so much but wasn't able to translate what I was learning to give back to him, at least in the short term. As I reflected more on our conversations, I realized that I was in fact providing a service in return. I was giving Mike a unique outlet to express himself and share his experiences. Furthermore, by increasing my appreciation of his lived experience with his condition, Mike was making me a better doctor and thus was using his experience to help give back to others.

This project has been a wonderful way for me to get to experience the unique intimacy that exists between doctors and their patients which is what brought me to medicine in the first place. My interest in the lived experience of illness and in using longitudinal relationships along with biomedical interventions to help care for patients is a driving force for my career in medicine. I am so grateful for and humbled by my experiences this year and I know that I will always carry the lessons I have learned with me.

UNDERSTANDING

Stories move in circles. They don't go in straight lines.
So it helps if you listen in circles.

— Sue Bender,
Everyday Sacred: A Woman's Journey Home

The Diagnosis

CLARE MALONE

At the age of 39, Giana was a healthy kindergarten teacher who had been teaching for close to 20 years in the Boston Public School system. In November, she went for her yearly mammogram, as she had been doing every year since she turned 25, due to a family history of breast cancer. This time was different though, because unlike every other mammogram, she got a phone call telling her that the results were abnormal. Giana went back for another mammogram in December and, again, in January, when they finally took a biopsy. Giana had breast cancer. For many women, at 39, this news would be surprising, but Giana had been expecting it at some level. Her mother, aunt, and sister had all been diagnosed with breast cancer before her. The doctor assured her that they caught her cancer early. Pathology revealed that she had ductal carcinoma in situ, or DCIS, the earliest stage of breast cancer. "It's a stage zero," the doctor told her, downplaying the fact that it was cancer.

Perhaps the doctor meant to reassure her, but Giana felt insulted by the way he dismissed her cancer. "Cancer is cancer, right?" she asked me. "I mean, I don't care if it's a stage zero, it is still cancer. It's still scary and it's still dangerous."

Her doctor advocated a lumpectomy followed by radiation, the standard treatment for DCIS. But Giana's mother had died of a radiation-induced tumor after she had a lumpectomy. "He thought I was over-reacting," she told me. "He kept saying that DCIS was stage zero and that I didn't need a mastectomy, so I found a different doctor who agreed with me." Giana had seen the power of breast cancer; she had lost her mother when she was just 4 years old, and she was not about to treat the enemy lightly. So Giana had a double mastectomy, followed by two rounds of reconstructive surgeries.

When Giana asked her doctor about the genetic factor—a mother and a sister with breast cancer before the age of 40 is difficult to overlook—they tested her for mutations in two breast cancer associated genes (*BRCA1* and *BRCA2*). She didn't have a mutation in either gene. "I guess your family is just really unlucky," the doctor told Giana. Giana was shocked at the cavalier way he wrote off her family's medical history. "I knew there was something genetic," she told me. "I knew we were not just unlucky."

So Giana became an expert in her family's medical history. She contacted aunts and cousins and carefully charted out her family tree, noting each mention of cancer. Once she collected all the information, it was painfully clear to her that her family wasn't "unlucky." There was something in their genes. Giana wanted a rational explanation for all of the cancer in her family; she wanted to know the gene responsible. So she went from genetic counselor to genetic counselor, family tree in hand, until finally one of them had a suggestion. He noticed that Giana's uncle had died of leukemia before the age of 30, and he realized that it might not be *breast* cancer that ran in the family, but any cancer. Most cancer predispositions predispose a patient to one or two specific types of cancer, not a wide range of cancers. But one incredibly rare syndrome is known to do just that, so the genetic counselor finally suggested testing for a mutation that could cause Li-Fraumeni syndrome. The genetic counselor warned Giana that Li-Fraumeni syndrome (LFS) is exceedingly rare. "You have a better chance of winning the lottery," he told her. But, nonetheless, when the test results came back they showed that Giana did, in fact, have Li-Fraumeni syndrome, a hereditary cancer syndrome. The occurrence of cancer in families with Li-Fraumeni syndrome is much higher than chance alone could explain. The overall lifetime cancer risk for a man with LFS is 73 percent. For women, the risk is close to 100 percent.

Through my talks with Giana, it has quickly become clear that her disease is much much more than the constellation of cancer diagnoses and surgeries listed on her medical chart. Even while cancer free, Giana and her family bore the scars of this disease, both literally and figuratively. Doctors generally take family medical histories in order to learn more about their patients' health, and in Giana's case her family history was critical for determining her eventual diagnosis.

But for Giana, her family medical history is so much more than this. A disease like Li-Fraumeni has particularly devastating effects on a family. When talking about having Li-Fraumeni, it is impossible for Giana to discuss only her own illness. When I first asked Giana to quite simply tell me about her medical history, she said, "It started before I was born." What she is referring to is the first moment that Li-Fraumeni started affecting her life, because her mother was first diagnosed with breast cancer when she was eight-months pregnant with Giana. The Li-Fraumeni story does not begin last May with a diagnosis, or even last January when Giana was first diagnosed with a cancer due to the syndrome. Instead, the story begins with Giana's mother's illness, because this has had a profound impact on Giana's life.

Giana's mother underwent a lumpectomy and, not knowing that she had Li-Fraumeni, had radiation treatment, and ultimately died when Giana was only four years old. This loss continues to stay with Giana. "I have a hole in my heart," she tells me, because she grew up without her mother. Because her mother was diagnosed with breast cancer while she was pregnant with Giana, she has always had feelings of guilt over her mother's death. She entered therapy at an early age to cope with these feelings.

The familial aspect of this disease carries huge weight for those who have it. On their biography pages at the Li-Fraumeni support group website, every single member makes reference to the mutation status of family members. Many members are the only people left in their family, and even more have decided not to have children because of the disease. Other members lost parents when they were small children, or their own children died at young ages. For the younger members, there is a lot of active discussion about the decision to have children or not, both out of fear of passing on the mutation and fear of dying young and leaving their children parentless.

LFS has also affected Giana's family planning, even before she knew she carried the mutation. Giana had a miscarriage when she was 36, and this loss has profoundly affected her. It's impossible to know whether LFS caused the miscarriage, although it has been suggested that women with LFS have higher rates of repetitive pregnancy loss. Unfortunately, in Giana's case, after her uterine lining was cleaned out to remove the miscarriage with a D & C (dilation and curettage or scraping)—which she had when the doctor told her that the pregnancy wasn't viable—some of the products of conception were left inside of her, which led to infection of her fallopian tubes, bleeding, and future fertility problems. After this, she and her husband looked into *in vitro* fertilization (IVF), where the egg is fertilized outside the body and then implanted in the uterus. They consulted a specialist who told them they were good candidates and that it was likely to be successful. However, Giana's husband decided that he was not comfortable moving forward with this, given Giana's family history of estrogen-positive breast cancer. He was worried that the hormones Giana would have to take in order to undergo *in vitro* fertilization might contribute to an acceleration of cancer, if she developed it.

Giana wanted a child desperately. This topic comes up again and again in our talks, and the look in her eyes when we talk about it suggests that her miscarriage also left "a hole in her heart." Giana tells me that she wants to adopt but that her husband isn't sure. "We are considering it," she says. But something about the way she says it tells me that she knows that she will probably never be a parent, and that this fact is one of the greatest sorrows in her life. Perhaps more important for Giana than the fact that LFS took away her breasts, her ovaries, and her uterus, LFS has decimated her family, and destroyed the chance she had to start a new family of her own.

I first met Giana at the end of a harrowing year: She had been diagnosed with breast cancer, had a double mastectomy, reconstructive surgery, learned that she had LFS, had a total hysterectomy, and had a growth removed from her colon. But she seemed upbeat and optimistic about her future, as if the worst was over. When I left the hospital that night, I had conflicting feelings. On the one hand, I could not help thinking how lucky Giana was. I had been bracing myself for a patient on death's doorstep, and here was a chatty, smiley, charming woman who appeared perfectly healthy. For a patient with Li-Fraumeni, she had done a remarkable job of catching her cancer and pre-cancerous lesions early, and had probably saved her own life by electing to undergo a double mastectomy rather than a lumpectomy followed by radiation, when she was diagnosed with DCIS. Radiation is extremely dangerous in patients with LFS, because it can easily cause a new tumor.

Giana points out that they have been much luckier than others with LFS. She and her sisters attended a convention for families with LFS this past year, and there she heard story upon story that made hers pale in comparison. There were people there with five or six active cancers. Others were fighting off their third cancer. Others had lost their parents at young ages, only to then watch helplessly as their children died at even younger ages. Still others are the only remaining living person in their family. The online support group for LFS tells similarly heart-wrenching stories. It's impossible to read the profiles without realizing the tragedies they have had to face time and time again in their lives, coupled with fear for their own health and the health of the few loved ones they have left. When you compare this with Giana, a healthy, active, and happy kindergarten teacher, happily married, she does seem to be lucky in some ways.

Giana says that she has often been accused of being a hypochondriac, but she has never been wrong about her body. "I just listen to my body," she tells me when I ask how she deals with the knowledge that she has LFS. "And if a doctor won't listen to me about my concerns, I find a new doctor." Giana says she is very careful with her health, and makes sure that anything that feels "off" is checked out by a doctor. While this diligent approach has kept her healthy so far, it has also made her quite overwhelmed. She has a file folder full of information about the various doctors she has seen over the last year and all of their opinions.

"The most difficult part is that there is no one person who keeps track of all of this for me; I have to be that one person," Giana tells me. She has seen countless doctors at nearly every Boston area hospital over the last few years, and each one records a portion of her story. But Giana herself is responsible for keeping track of her records, knowing what tests she has had done, and how she can get the images and results when another doctor requests them.

For Giana, one of the worst days of her life was long before her diagnosis of Li-Fraumeni. Giana and her husband were trying to have a baby, and she was finally pregnant, much to their delight. But at a routine visit to the obstetrician, her doctor told her that her baby was not viable. He recommended a Dilation and Curettage (D&C) of the uterus to remove the dead tissue, and told her that without it she would miscarry naturally anyway. She consented to the D&C. A few days later, while her husband was at work and she was with a female friend, Giana began to hemorrhage. She was rushed to the hospital and her friend elected to ride in the ambulance with her, so that she was not alone.

"I'm Russian orthodox, so I wear my wedding ring on my right hand," Giana tells me. "Maybe they thought I wasn't married and that I had an abortion, because I didn't want the baby." She thinks for a minute and then continues, "I was also with a female friend when I started to hemorrhage, and she rode in the ambulance with me to the hospital. I don't know, maybe the doctor thought I was a lesbian." We both sit for a minute pondering these possibilities, thinking about whether they can explain her doctor's behavior. Maybe I am overestimating my powers of deduction, but I think I can tell that we have come to the same conclusion. Nothing explains this doctor's behavior. Giana was hemorrhaging as a result of products of conception being left behind after a D & C. It doesn't matter why Giana had the D & C, who Giana was married to, or whether she was married at all. This would be a scary and difficult time for anyone, and a doctor should respect that and care for her patient in way that demonstrates empathy.

At the hospital, a tall, blond, beautiful doctor was assigned to Giana's case. Giana did not give me specifics, but she said the doctor treated her very coldly, and in a very abrupt manner. She did not doctor Giana's emotional wounds at all. There was also a young intern there, a nerdy doctor with glasses and a yalmulka. He did not have the glamour of his attending, but he did have a heart. When he dealt with Giana he was gentle and showed an understanding of how she might be feeling.

While in the hospital, Giana learned that the baby she had lost, whom she still refers to as her baby, was a girl. This piece of information made the loss of her child so much more real. Giana and her husband had already picked out a name if they had a daughter, and now to Giana it really felt like she had lost a child—a daughter.

This would have been a sad day for Giana regardless of who her doctor was, but, perhaps, her pain could have been a little lighter if she had not also felt that her doctor was judging her and cared very little about helping her. For the doctor, Giana was probably just one of many patients that she saw that day, and with the hemorrhaging stopped and the remaining products of conception removed, the doctor felt her job was done.

Giana tells me that she later pulled aside the young, nerdy intern who had been kind to her, and told him not to become a doctor like his boss, because, as she said, "I will never let that woman put her hands on me again."

Over lunch, Giana asks me more about the project. What exactly do I have to write up? Who am I sharing this with? I tell her more about the project, and about how most of the people in the class are actually future doctors rather than scientists. "Will you tell them something for me?" Giana asks. I say, "Of course." Her message is simple: Patients are people with feelings and emotions, and a good doctor will never forget that, not for one moment. Even if it's the thousandth time you have diagnosed someone with a particular disease, it is always the first time for the patient.

Infinity

DANIEL SEIBLE

"I have some bad news."

"Is Daddy going to die?"

"No."

"Then it can't be bad news."

"He's going to lose his other arm . . . about here."

"Oh, that's nothing. It doesn't matter if Daddy has no arms or legs . . . as long as he's alive, then I still have my dad."

Katherine still revels in her eight-year-old son's profound insight into what truly matters in life. But this story is more about Jeff Van Kempen, aka "Daddy." I met Jeff on a cool, fall evening in the burn ward. I was fresh into my first year at Harvard Medical School, and had signed up for an elective course tailored to learning about "the patient experience." The course matched me up with a burn surgeon and one of his patients, whom I would follow throughout the year.

Walking into the burn ward was humbling. As I waited about 45 minutes for the resident surgeon to return from the OR and introduce me to Mr. Van Kempen, I looked around and saw some of the most horrendous medical disfigurations imaginable. Before that day, I would see a teenager with acne or a patient in a wheelchair and wonder about how it must be hard for them to interact in society. After one tour of the burn unit, every other visible ailment paled in comparison. To think I even looked twice at the patch of hair that wouldn't quite lie flat on the back of my head that morning made me feel dirty with superficial vanity. I waited near reception and began to become more nervous about what sort of first impression I would leave on Jeff.

Finally, Dr. Frank, the burn resident for the month of October, returned from the OR and sat me down to talk about what I was there for. My official mentor was out of town and had delegated the introduction to the resident on duty. Dr. Frank explained that the patient, Jeff Van Kempen, had worked on power lines as a profession, and was badly burned on the job a few weeks before. Apparently, while on a cherry-picker platform, something went awry, and Jeff fell onto active wires on both his right and left sides and upper arms. After initial stabilization to several attempts at debridement (excision of tissue damaged by the burns), the onset of a life-threatening infection resulted in the amputation of first one arm and then the other, to save Jeff's life. Dr. Frank had been taking care of Jeff for most of the time he had been in the hospital, and was optimistic about the mutual benefit Jeff and I might experience. After Dr. Frank checked with Jeff about the timing of my visit, and reassured him that I was definitely not a Yankees fan, we walked down the hall to Jeff's room.

I met Jeff while he was sitting in a chair next to his hospital bed watching a baseball game. My hands always sweat profusely when I am nervous, and I was wiping my palms on my pants to avoid an awkwardly moist handshake, when I realized, feeling quite silly, that shaking hands was not in order when meeting a person who had lost both of his. Jeff is a tall man in his prime: 40 years old, happily married, father to both an eight-year-old son and a five-year-old daughter. Jeff's wife, Katherine, who popped in for the second half of our meeting, had a warm personality and a determined optimism about her that showed through her ready smile and comforting small talk. Jeff and I went through casual introductions, and I shared a bit about what life was like for me, moving with my wife from Southern California to New England to start medical school. Jeff was polite and open to answering any of my questions, which I kept fairly general to ease into our first time together. Jeff was very much determined to get out of the hospital and into rehabilitation—and back to life. He hadn't seen his kids since before the accident, as he had decided, with Katherine, that it might be too soon for their young children to process. He obviously missed them dearly. Although open and alert, Jeff never once smiled during the conversation, and I don't blame him. If I were just starting to digest the ramifications of losing both arms and almost my life to an accident, I'd have a hard time smiling too.

At one time during the conversation with the Van Kempen family, I tried out the perennial mantra of medical student interviewing skills—"This must be hard for you"—and was shocked by their response of "Actually, it has been much better than we would ever expect. The doctors are amazing, and our friends, family and neighbors have been incredibly supportive. Even the kids are handling it really well." If anyone deserves to respond with "Yes, actually, it is horribly difficult," it would be them.

Jeff shared an interesting memory: "*I distinctly remember a woman named Celeste kneeling by the hospital bed listing all the reasons I wasn't going to make it.*"

Celeste is an intriguing character. One might wonder what kind of sick-minded person would kneel next to the critically injured to deliver a litany of reasons they were going to die. Evidently, Celeste doesn't work at the hospital and she isn't a nurse, doctor, or clergywoman. Who is this mysteriously sinister person, you ask? As far as Jeff and Katherine know, neither of them even knows a woman named Celeste. She turns out to be a hallucination of Jeff's, during the first few days of coming around after his accident. Surprisingly, a large number of burn patients on ventilators have at least one delirious episode during recovery. To this day, Jeff struggles to recall the murky details of his revival after the extensive surgeries he underwent following the accident, but he clearly recalls the imaginary encounter with Celeste, the phantom herald of malady.

On one visit, I stumbled into a meeting between Jeff, Katherine, their two children, and two of Jeff's coworkers, who were finally given permission to visit Jeff and wish him well. From the start it was obvious that Jeff's two middle-aged female associates were deeply moved by his resilience in the face of hardship. They recounted the circumstances of hearing about the accident, and how emotional repercussions rippled through Jeff's workplace after word got out. Jeff was very well liked and respected on the job, and a majority of the visit was spent fondly recalling how a fellow lineman named Mike tried day after day to visit Jeff, and once successfully gaining permission, repeatedly delivered unhealthy but welcome snacks to his bedridden comrade.

Jeff graduated ahead of schedule from the burn ward into the Rehabilitation Hospital. It was obvious that tremendous physical and emotional recovery took place since last we spoke, as Jeff no longer had breathing assistance and was sitting and standing unaided without much difficulty. Most impressively to me, Jeff now wore an intermittent smile that permeated the solemnity of his situation, and brought rays of joy into his family's faces at each emergence. The bedridden and wearily polite man I met just 14 days before had undergone tremendous healing in more ways than one. Beside the bright red marks on his thighs from the donor sites of his previous skin grafts, it was almost easy to forget I was talking to an acutely ill person.

Earlier that day, Jeff was casted for the future fitting of a prosthetic arm over the remainder of his right-upper extremity. He was not sure what extent of functionality it would provide, but was looking forward to gaining back his independence in basic hygiene. Katherine lovingly joked about her fears of shaving Jeff's face, which were escalated when the attending physician humorously quipped, "Oh, and make sure you don't cut him because of the heparin!" Heparin is a blood thinner many people are dosed with during extensive healing due to the risk of blood clots breaking off and clogging essential arteries. As nice as levity is in some tense situations, I'm not sure the quip eased Katherine's nerves when it came to helping her husband shave. Talking with Jeff and his wife made me appreciate the autonomy I take for granted on a daily basis. I happily rely on my wife for a few small things, such as remembering where anything and everything I've lost happens to be. However, I can now imagine how difficult and frustrating it is for a patient who is used to personal agency in mundane functions to cope with the reality of an unexpected dependency.

"Galen has become almost a little man-boy, trying to take care of his sister and mom."

"You must be very proud."

"I am, I really am."

It was the closest I'd seen Jeff to tearing up. There had been times where he seemed shaken by the profundity of his physical loss, but talking about how his son has been growing up before his eyes, to help the family in a time of stress, was deeply moving to him. Jeff said the absolute worst part of the accident was that he felt his injury's burden on his family. "I obviously didn't ask for this, but I can handle losing my arms. It's seeing all the little things my family will have to do for me while I regain autonomy that is really difficult," he reflected, when asked what the hardest part of the ordeal was. Jeff and Katherine's five-year-old daughter, Haley, was having a difficult time from her dad's extended absence, and was frequently in tears. The weight of her sadness was added incentive to an already determined and optimistic man. It was obvious that Jeff was giving his all to the multiple occupational therapy and rehabilitation sessions that comprised his daily schedule at the Rehabilitation Center.

Despite the lingering burdens of trauma, I realized that Jeff smiled even more than the previous visit. It was exciting to see the raw human spirit of what must have been the good-humored man I hadn't met before the accident. Strangely, I felt lucky to have come into Jeff's life at such a low point. Unlike his family, friends, neighbors and coworkers, who saw steady progression back to the great man they knew, I had the opportunity to meet someone in a time of hardship, confusion, and pain. There was nowhere to go but up, and I was privileged to witness Jeff's ascent. It was positively inspiring to meet a person in such disarray build a happy life out of the chaos of sudden illness. Jeff even mentioned dreams of possibly using his experience and story to help educate younger linemen about the dangers of the profession and the necessity of diligence on the job. That inclination, combined with Jeff's openness in agreeing to have an untrained, strange medical student chronicle his intimate and difficult experience, speak volumes about his generous spirit. I've already learned so much from Jeff Van Kempen, it is certain that he will make an enormous impact in the lives of many to come.

Because Jeff was working for a company with good benefits during his accident, he does not have to worry as much about the financial burden of the circumstance. "A huge part of my quick recovery has been a feeling of being taken care of," Jeff reflected, "and I don't think I would feel that way if I had to worry about my family struggling without my income." It was an obvious point of relief, and Jeff constantly added how lucky he was to have what so many people are left without after grievous accidents. Overwhelmed with Jeff's infectious optimism and gratitude, I nervously ventured a question as to if he saw any unexpected good in the experience. Without hesitation, Jeff replied that he was looking at life in a new and positive way. Although he spent time with his family before, even coaching his kids' sports teams, he was a very busy person without much down time. He now looks forward to being around his kids after school and during other times, where he otherwise wouldn't have had the opportunity were it not for the accident.

During that meeting, I worked in a little bit of a medical history for the sake of completeness. Unsurprisingly, being a healthy 40-year-old man, Jeff's laundry list of medical history was more of a Post-It note. While at this point he was still taking blood pressure pills, antibiotics, pain medications, and iron supplements, before the accident Jeff was on nothing. He exercised regularly in the gym and refereed sporting events, and had an almost spotless bill of health. Beside a slight heart arrhythmia, difficulty swallowing food from time to time, some ear tubes as a child, and a benign toe growth removed in his twenties, Jeff was the picture of health. Even just a few weeks post-accident, he looked healthier than most 40-year-old men.

Jeff reported pain only during the rigorous stretching program that is part of his rehabilitation, but felt extreme frustration with "phantom" sensation in his amputated arms. "It is a horribly frustrating feeling," Jeff explained, "knowing my arms aren't there but still having total sensation." Phantom pain is discomfort associated with a body part that's no longer there. This was once thought to be purely psychological, but experts now think that these sensations originate in the spinal cord and brain, because the control center in the brain is still intact and causes phantom sensations to persist. Jeff felt his right hand closed into a fist, and no matter what he did or how he rotated his remaining shoulder and stub, he could not change the sensation. He described the feeling as surreal, almost like being paralyzed but having total sensation at the same time.

Jeff was definitely anxious and eager to get home. "What's the hardest part of it all?"

"It's all about the kids and Katherine. I put my family in this position of living without a dad and a husband. I feel the only way I can help out is to come home. "

When I arrived, Jeff was out for a round of physical therapy, and I had a chance to talk to Katherine, Jeff's sister, and Jeff's boss, who were all there waiting to visit. All three were glowing with pride for their loved one. Jeff's boss was enthusi- astically talking about charity events they were planning to benefit the family, and the atmosphere of the room was brim- ming with optimism. The positive energy was enough that Katherine was able to recount the two occasions that physi- cians had told her she would probably lose her husband in the night, without stirring up emotions in the story telling. Beside having a release date to look forward to, Jeff was excelling at occupational therapy tasks, such as feeding himself with a strap apparatus and pulling his pants up and down with a pole- and-hook device rigged up by his therapist.

Jeff taught me that, although many buildings are "handi- capped accessible," they cater mainly to a specific subset of physically challenged, namely those confined to wheel chairs but who have normal arm function. However, the physically impaired come in many more flavors, of which Jeff is living proof. Stairs provide no obstacle to Jeff, who at this stage in re- covery can traverse multiple flights without breaking a sweat. A doorknob, on the other hand, seems insurmountable. Wheel- chair ramps and bars to help maneuver a public restroom do people like Jeff almost no good at all. Buttons to push for open- ing doors are not designed to activate using a hip. These are only a few examples that many people, including myself, never thought about before meeting someone like Jeff. For Jeff, and other people like him, these structures become serious bar- riers between a person and their place in a functional society.

Jeff was very excited about his impending prosthesis-fit- ting and therapy, and mentioned he expected his skin to be mostly healed in about a month. He also said that a surgeon in the area had contacted him. wanting to talk about the idea of an arm transplant operation. Although there have been some successful hand and arm transplantations, up to 85 percent of the patients experienced at least one episode of acute rejection during the first year post-transplant, and complications of immune suppression included opportunistic infections, metabolic complications, and malignancies. Jeff was thinking he probably wouldn't be interested in such a dangerous procedure still in its infancy, but would still schedule a meeting with the surgeon to hear him out.

Before leaving, Katherine gave me access to an online program called "Care Pages." It is a system that allows messages to be posted to concerned friends and family about a patient's status, and also provides a forum for outsiders to post words of encouragement to the family and patient. I asked Jeff about whether it made a difference in his recovery. "Oh, God, yes!" he replied. "If you go on, it will show you that there are 700 people signed up to view updates. Before looking at my Care Page, I didn't even think I knew 700 people, let alone think I had that many people care about me." After returning home after that visit, I created an account, and used the information Katherine gave me to look Jeff up. The resilience of Katherine's optimism and the response of Jeff's loved ones were impressive. Words of love and encouragement effervesced around each update, and every reply was a caring act of raw humanity.

"What's it like being an inpatient for over a month?"

"It's infinity. I mean, you're not a prisoner, but then again you are. I'll be happy if I never see a hospital for the rest of my life."

My last time visiting Jeff as an inpatient, I'd expected to see him and Katherine exuberant about his upcoming "release" to the world outside of hospitals. Both were tired of waiting, to be sure; however, Jeff had developed a severe bowel infection, which caused diarrhea and delayed his discharge from the hospital. Besides having diarrhea for a couple of days, Jeff also was started on a new blood pressure medication that he couldn't swallow. Furthermore, the long-awaited prosthetic arm was late in arriving. After all the family had been through, last minute complications were the last thing they needed. Mountains of paperwork awaited Jeff and Katherine at home, and both seemed to feel a little apprehensive about what life would be like back at home.

"Are you excited?" I asked, thinking of the release date only a few days off. "Yes, but apprehensive as well. I'm worried that times will come where I won't be able to do something for my kids." Previously, I had been thinking about how great it would be if I were Jeff, to finally get back to my family and life outside of the hospital. I hadn't thought about how drastic a change it would be to come back to a life with an old, established role that I couldn't immediately fill. If my child were nearby and had fallen, I couldn't walk over and pick her up. If kids needed help to get ready, and my wife wasn't around, how would I help them? Presence, it occurs to me while writing, is not sufficient when considering a return to life. The life of a spectator is not the same. Knowing Jeff's work ethic and determination, he will surely find creative ways to sidestep the hurdles of disability. However, this process will have a steep learning curve, which would take anyone, even the most imaginative and energetic people, quite a while to master.

Additionally, Jeff knows that life in a small town, where everyone is very much aware of his accident, will unavoidably be different. He isn't sure how things will change, but is concerned that people will feel compelled to treat "Jeff since the accident" differently than "our friend Jeff." Wisely, Jeff and Katherine have requested a few days respite after returning home, before waves of well-wishers descend on their home. Although an occupational therapist has been helping Jeff work on opening doors and changing clothes independently, the time he was hoping to work on skills with his prosthesis will now have to wait for later outpatient visits. As I spoke with Jeff, Katherine was on her new tablet (a recent gift from family), looking up lever-based doorknobs and towel-less bathroom dryer systems. Jeff wondered about working for the company that sells the systems, since their past spokesperson was an amputee with a similar story. He also had plans to start coaching basketball again, as early as a couple of weeks from discharge. Routine, as Jeff frequently alluded to, will be a theme in his recovery. He hoped to have enough planned throughout the day to keep him busy and on the mend, both physically and emotionally.

Katherine sent me an email update once they were home again:

> *Dan,*
>
> *Things are going well as far as a nursing, physical therapy, and occupational therapy perspective. We have felt the transition was flawless and in sync with the same expectations that the rehabilitation staff would have had if we choose an outpatient care through them. Jeff is adjusting as best he can. Still no computer or phone for him to be able to use, so a bit frustrating on that end with Workman's Comp. We did finally receive the arm on Friday, however, Friday evening Jeff developed a blister on one of his skin grafts in the back, so due to having to put a brace on that side, we are unable to use and practice with his arm. So a few setbacks have become quite a large obstacle for Jeff. I will keep you posted as to how things go over the next couple weeks and let you know when we have an appt in Boston after the 1st of the year.*
>
> *Katherine and Jeff*

Jeff's experience highlights the fact that a falsely positive projection of future events can set a patient up for failed expectations. Negative reaction comes quickly to any person whose expectations of the future are not met, and among the challenged-patient population this rings particularly true. As a future representative of the healthcare system, I will certainly try to be mindful when telling a patient when to expect an intervention or positive outcome. Alternatively, I will also need to be aware of the devastation an overly-conservative estimation can cause to a patient and their family. While Jeff was in a critical state in the burn ward, Katherine endured multiple conversations with physicians telling her that Jeff would probably not make it through the night. Medicine is a mix of balance, grey areas, and pitfalls. Perhaps it is because life is messy, people are complex, and physicians tend to enter into people's lives at the messiest parts.

Knowing Jeff and seeing the healing he experiences in having positive goals and working toward them in a structured way, I am certain the weeks of waiting past the expected date to receive his prosthesis became a mammoth challenge of the man's patience. Every time I visited Jeff in the hospital or rehabilitation, he could quickly recall the exact number of days the doctors had told him to expect to endure at each care facility. The one relief of seemingly unbearable waiting is hope that the end point will come. Luckily, Jeff worked hard and was ahead of schedule on his transfer to rehabilitation and later release to home. But when the day of expected prosthesis arrival came and went, the imagined schedule of improvement, by which Jeff measures proactive healing, was marred. When that day turned into a week, and then two, I'm sure Jeff was revisited by his ghost of timeless paralysis, which he knew so well when waiting for discharge from rehabilitation.

What, then, is the role of a physician in helping a patient visualize his or her future? Is it to encourage and give hope? Should doctors, instead, give a pessimistic, conservative estimate, so the patient is not discouraged by setbacks? Physicians could be tempted to shirk the practice of prognosis altogether and avoid the emotional rollercoaster of surpassing or failing expectations. However, to do so would be to deny patients the humanity of whole-person care. A patient's perception of his or her future has long been proven to be a significant factor in healing, and, as such, deserves physician time and attention. Thus, as a doctor, I will strive to use what I've learned about the significance of a physician's predictions, to help me navigate the intricacies of helping people understand the future of their condition.

Jeff continued to correspond with me on a regular basis:

Dan,

Adjusting to life at home has actually not been that bad. I find as long as I just have patience that I will be able to figure out things that I need to figure out. It is still frustrating to have to ask for things to be done for you as it just doesn't seem fair to ask your kids and your wife to do things that I should be able to do if this had not happened to me. The prosthetic arm I have has been nothing short of a source of frustration for me as it in no way added anything to my life. That is probably a harsh statement but it seems with what I've been given to work with just does not do anything for me. Although I have not given up on it I will continue to work and hopefully in the future it might help me the way that they think it should.

The things that have surprised me in a good way are that there are so many people who are willing to help. The people in this community and my friends in the local area have been great. From the committee who set up a fundraiser in my honor and raised $18,000 for my family and all of the help we've been given from people plowing out our driveway to overall support has been nothing short of greatness. I am also very happy with the therapy I have been given at the local rehab hospital. They really seem to care about me and it is something that I look forward to attending three times a week.

245

The things that have surprised me in a bad way are more things that psychologically I think about. For example, just watching how life continues and how I am on the sidelines. I know that this is totally out of my control for now, but only four months having been removed from my normal life you already feel that you have been forgotten about. Another thing that has surprised me is the lack of visitation from people far away, but again I guess it would be unfair for me to think that everyone should just drop everything and come visit me. Don't get me wrong. I have had more than a few visitors but it just seems that more of my relatives would want to see me as well as friends. But people do have their own lives and I have to realize that I am not the center of those lives. I think probably everyone will have that point in their lives where they feel isolated but I have experienced mine a little sooner than most.

The most frustrating thing is not being able to pick up anything or help with anything. But I know one time that I will get a little bit better. One of the things that has happened is that I have purchased a new car that will be outfitted with foot steering and hopefully after driver training I can pass my driver examination and get my license back. This will allow me at least a little more freedom.

As far as the ice and snow I just have to take it easy when walking and as far as my balance goes the physical therapists are really amazed at my balance.
Take care

Jeff

After receiving this email from Jeff, I pondered how true his words ring with many walks of life, and I gained new perspective on the phenomenon of attention swings in times of personal drama. The humility of self-realization is rarely provoked more profoundly than when we lose the attention that follows major changes in life. A pet dies, a loved-one is diagnosed with an illness, a possession is lost, and we see friends and family giving us extra consideration and love to make up for our loss. Conversely, in times of happiness, all the same people come alongside you to share in your joy. After the all-too-short honeymoon of cooperative jubilation or love-soaked sympathy, reality strikes hard. Your dog does not come back to life or your family member is still chronically ill. You face the consequences of the provocative drama a little more alone, or, at least, as alone as you were before the excitement. Your life is changed for better or for worse, but also now the extended network of humanity that answers to the transient trumpet of change has receded to its normal day-to-day. A glimmer of hope remains for the diligent, though. You see your smaller circles of family and friends for the support-structure they are. You realize the worth in virtues like patience, and you learn to rely on the recently less-than-fully-appreciated copilots of your life. You find fulfillment in plodding through the endless tunnel of work and learning, to which you have (either willfully or compulsively) entered. For Jeff, he can only react to the medical phenomenon that snatched him out of his livelihood.

According to research sponsored by the Landmine Survivors Network, victims of sudden limb loss require multifaceted support for productive psychological recovery. Of influences relative to such recovery, the most important were "the individual's resilience characteristics, social support, medical care, economic situation and societal attitudes toward people with disabilities." Luckily, social support is only one factor of many, and Jeff is quite blessed with a loving family and friend network. Regardless, it is that which changes quickly that we notice most heavily, and a retraction of enormous social support would be difficult for anyone to process.

As a physician, I would do well to remember that the patients for whom I am caring did not ask for illness. They did not inspect the universe of medicine, as I did, and think "Hmm, this is interesting and difficult, but I think I will give it a go." People like Jeff would like nothing better than to healthily evade hospitals for the remainder of their lives. And although we have amazing networks of support that will rally to us in extreme times of personal chaos, for most of life you are surrounded, instead, by your own thoughts—and, of course, those friends and family who were just as interested in loving you before the chaos as afterward.

Dan,

As far as the computer goes, I have a new laptop with the Dragon software installed that I'm using now to draft this e-mail. In addition to that, I have a foot operated mouse with a foot operated pedal, which allows me to navigate everything I need.

As far as using my legs or feet, I actually do minimal things with them other than opening a door, or using my computer like I mentioned above or occasionally operating the remote control. I also use my feet for other various things throughout the day but it is not a huge part of my daily routine.

I have been able to spend a lot of time with my family, which has been a bonus. However, it seems that my relationship with my kids is somewhat different. And they do view me differently, which is very difficult. I know as they grow older, this will slowly disappear as it must be very difficult for them to deal with. As far as pursuing interests, I have found getting into family genealogy is very interesting, as long as doing a lot of reading on the computer, which I never seemed to have time for before.

As far as daily structure goes I am up in the morning helping getting the kids ready for school and once they leave at around eight o'clock in the morning. I exercise for about 1 1/2 hours. After that I spent about an hour and a half on the computer and then watched television until lunchtime when the occupational therapist comes into my home and we prepare lunch and then do other household things that may help me. Usually by this time is around 1:30. I do a few exercises spend a little time at the computer, maybe take a nap and by this time the kids and Katherine are home and we start our nighttime routine. This will probably change when the better weather comes as I will be able to spend more time outside. Hopefully within four months I will have my driver's license, which will add to my independence.

Off the record, having been five months after this happened many things really start to occur to you. One is that you are nothing but a total drain on everybody else. Secondly, nobody will ever view you as an equal. People seem to look at you and you can tell the expression on their faces that they are just thinking to themselves, Boy I'm glad that's not me. Don't get me wrong. People are very supportive. But I guess it's just up to me to just live out the string and do the best that I can because of my wife and kids. One thing is for sure. I have to motivate myself or it is just not going to happen.

I do have a lot of things to be thankful for, but living like this is certainly not one of them.
Take care.

Jeff"

Mulling over Jeff's words, I came across a startling revelation. This type of objectifying people by their physical appearance is rampant in medicine. Luckily, steps are being made to address this tendency to reduce patients to their illnesses. In medical school, we have had a few discussions about awareness that a patient is more than a diagnosis, more than pathology, more than the machine we've been trained to fix. However, we necessarily have had many, many more conversations about biochemistry, anatomy, and physiology. For a long while, in medical education it was assumed that life prior to medicine taught you how to respect and treat the human aspect of a patient. It is a good thing steps are being made to account for the fact that many new students of medicine have much more experience solving scientific problems than they do sympathizing with the ill.

To Jeff, some friends and acquaintances no longer see him as the active husband, father, and person he used to be. He can now be seen in the light of being "the disabled person I know" to others. I'm not surprised this transition and realization has been difficult for Jeff, and I've no idea how Jeff will work through such a transition. Thankfully, with some technological advances, such as adaptive communications systems, which Jeff has at home, some of the smaller barriers to everyday life can be overcome with effort. Increasingly used in the home-based setting, software like Dragon's voice-recognition computer system has entered the personal computer industry, and adapts to the user's vocabulary and style of speech. While stylistically different from the average person's interaction with computing, advances such as this take a little disability away from the label of "disabled."

I remember that, as an adolescent, I visited an ophthalmologist about the eye-movement disorder I was born with. Although slight, it causes me to have a small head-turn when looking forward, and I was considering surgical correction. That day, the ophthalmologist said to me, "I can't make you perfect, but I can make you better." I remember the strange feeling of realizing that, in that moment, I *was* my disorder in the eyes of my ophthalmologist. He did not say "I can make your eyes better, but not perfect;" instead, it was "I can make *you* better."

The biggest problem with this tendency of humans to define reality by what is physically seen is that, when you see a person as a physical being, any lack or disturbance in physical normalcy is not just a disability. As Jeff wisely observed, it is an attack on your individual humanity. It makes the ill or disabled less than whole. If being a man is defined physically to people as having muscular arms and legs and a certain amount of weight and height, then someone who is confined to a chair is only half a man, vertically speaking. Or someone who lost twenty-five pounds of arms is twenty-five pounds less of a person.

Equality, in the deepest sense, will always be a struggle for the physically disabled, unless society is trained, and rigorously shown, to realize the assumptions our brains make every day, so that we might overcome them. Jeff and Katherine's children will learn those lessons growing up with a disabled father, but children who have no such personal experience may grow up only to think to themselves, upon encountering a disabled person, "Boy, I'm glad that's not me."

> *As far as dreams go, I don't recall really dreaming about it, but I do think a lot about it which probably isn't productive at all. Just thinking about if I had moved 1 inch differently. I wouldn't be in this situation. Not knowing exactly what happened is probably the worst thing. I still do have phantom pain from my arms, but the pain is always different. Sometimes you feel your hands more and sometimes you just feel the weight of the arms. But mostly I think that over time, you just start living with it. So one does not notice it as much.*

The rollercoaster of emotions that Jeff has needed to process over the last few months is more than I can understand. Some hurts, like phantom pains, he can combat with patience and time. Other injuries, deeper hurts, like the tapering off of emotional support from those who worked with Jeff before his accident, can instead inflame with duration. Pivotal negative experiences naturally grow into regret and doubt if left unchecked. Although Jeff is probably the most resilient man I've met, it can't be easy for him to suppress the instinct to play the timeless game of "what if." I consider myself an eternal optimist, but to reflect honestly, if I had been through what Jeff had, these thoughts would have surfaced sooner than six months after the incident.

Journalist Gary Stix wrote that resilience has been shown to be more prevalent in the general population than previously expected, but that certain post-traumatic reactions, such as "self-enhancing bias"—a self-perception similar to narcissism—actually help people to stave off negative rumination. Seeing Jeff interact with his family, and knowing that his dedication to recovery is not out of self-pity, but, instead, a desire to regain function in order to help, could actually be posing a challenge to resilience. If narcissism is, indeed, a common tool for those who cope with difficult recoveries, as suggested by Stix, it could naturally be difficult for Jeff to avoid the lure of negative thinking, due to his own quality of selflessness.

Many of the frustrations we suppress in life come out in difficult times of transition. From personal experience, I know I am more likely to complain about small things that frustrate me if I am having a bad day or something troubling is on my mind. These small things are not worth addressing normally, but in the heat of difficulty I lose the filter that tells me to let it go, because, in reality, it is so small. In like fashion, the negative memories of Jeff's workplace are now given free rein to resurface in this time of difficulty. I can imagine Jeff, with much more time to think and reflect than he's ever had, mulling over the situation in frustration, and having those small frustrations overwhelm him in his pain.

Thinking I have any chance of having a normal life again is just not realistic.

In the spring, I pulled my car up to Jeff and Katherine's lovely family home. It was a wonderful respite to tour a picturesque neighborhood, after a long morning of lectures; and I sat with windows open for a few minutes, to enjoy the spring weather. Jeff and Katherine's house was a beautiful, two-story home with a large, well-kept yard in the middle of a wide cul-de-sac. Soon, Jeff came down the street from walking his son to a play date, and led me into his home to catch up.

We sat for a few minutes in the living room with their friendly dog, Cali, exchanging small talk. Soon, Jeff started speaking about how he had a release surgery in March, to allow greater movement of his right shoulder, and how they were looking into a new procedure called TMR for Targeted Muscle Re-innervation. TMR is a procedure that reinserts the nerves of the arm into chest muscles, and allows patients to control their artificial limbs with these newly innervated muscles. Those signals from these muscles direct hand movement by using the same nerve that had originally been used to do so. While Jeff may be an ideal candidate for this technology, it remains to be seen to what extent insurance would cover the procedure, and if the promises of new technology actually pan out. While Jeff remains optimistic, his optimism has matured into an interest without expectation, a lesson hard-learned by hopes that were unmet with his current artificial limb.

Jeff described his current situation as still very frustrating, especially when he sees the toll it takes on Katherine. Beyond working thirty hours per week, Katherine now picks up all the chores that had been Jeff's responsibility prior to the accident. He also notes how difficult it must be for her to have almost no time to herself. Talking to Katherine confirmed the fatigue of the new adjustment, but beyond looking a little tired, the house was in immaculate order, and the family was obviously well cared for.

Small adjustments were still in process at the Van Kempen household, mainly the switching out of all knobbed controllers to lever-style handles. Jeff deftly navigates the web with his foot-operated computer, and the upstairs bathroom is outfitted with a hands-free body air-dryer. Beyond such small changes, the house would be indistinguishable from that of any other family. Jeff's current prosthesis allows him to do certain things, such as signing forms more easily than he could without it, but he still generally prefers to leave it off. The arm did, however, allow me to shake Jeff's hand for the first time after he put the arm on, and, again, when I left his home, which made me feel as though I connected with him on a more personal level. I wondered what it was like for him to experience a handshake without sensation.

Before leaving the Van Kempen home, Jeff and I chatted about productive things he could do, while he waited for the legal settlement to come to a close. Jeff would like to read more without being online, but it will take some time before he would be able to turn pages on a tablet using a stylus, due to prosthetic limitations. Seeing him navigate his computer so aptly got me thinking about computer-based learning modules, and I asked him if he had ever considered learning a language using computer-based software such as Rosetta Stone. Within a few minutes, I could see Jeff's mind at work, thinking of possibilities of contributing to his family financially as an interpreter. To me, it seemed the first time during the afternoon that the optimistic energy I remember seeing in him before began shining through the layered frustration. Jeff is definitely a man who thrives on productive, goal-oriented activity. I hope that he will soon be able to find his niche in this new, if not normal, life.

Dan,

I can't really think of anything about the medical system that I would like to change, the only thing that I can think of is that the easier you can make it for the patient the better. Obviously nobody likes to make the patient ever wait for anything, but the less a patient ever has to wait the better because nobody wants to think that their time is not important.

If I were addressing a room full of medical students, the first thing I would say is that I would want my doctor to be the best in their field every day. If someone isn't willing to strive for that then maybe this field is not for them. I realize not everyone can have great people skills, but human compassion obviously is very important, and striving to have that should never end.

My experience in this situation has taught me that life can take many different directions, so that no matter what happens, you have to make adjustments to make the most of any situation that you find yourself in. If you can do this, most things will come out in a good way. On the other hand, I have found that if something happens to you, it does not take long for everyone to move on without you. People have their own lives to lead and you just have to realize not to take this personally.

Surprisingly, my priorities have not really changed that much. My goal in life has always been to provide the best possible life for my family and make it as easy as possible for my kids and my wife. Although the situation has not helped, I find that my goal is still the same and that the only difference is that it's just a little slower pace.

I know that these are pretty plain answers, but I have to keep things simple as possible for myself. The only thing I'm struggling with right now is that I have a

lot of pent up hatred for a certain few people. I've never really experienced this in my life but I can tell you it is a horrible feeling, consuming at times. I have to find ways to not let this affect other areas of my life but it is diffi-cult sometimes. However, I am working on it.
Hope this helps,

Jeff

Wrapping up the year of following Jeff, I take to heart his advice for me to strive to be the best in my field and to intentionally grow my human compassion. While it is impossible for every doctor to be the best, it is well worth my attention to realize that, regardless of plausibility, the expectation of my patients for my abilities will be nothing short of excellence. I will aim for being the best in my field, but, at a minimum, I will not settle for less than my personal best for every patient, every day. As far as compassion, taking the extra time to get to know a patient beyond his or her illness has proven invaluable, with respect to insight into the human condition. I learned very little "conventional medicine" in my conversations with Jeff and his family, but what I did learn rivals the entirety of my first year's curriculum, in terms of application for my future practice of medicine.

I learned that communities have the potential to band together and make a healing difference in the life of a patient, but also that close friends and families are much more important for longterm recovery.

I learned that a patient's perception of the foreseeable future is inseparable from his or her current state of being, and that a physician's prognosis will greatly influence this.

I learned that illness and injury are as difficult for loved ones as they can be for patients, and that the committed love of a spouse is more valuable than health and stronger than any disease.

I learned that radiating resilience proves to be as much a productive addition to a family as completing any number of practical tasks.

I learned that the words a physician chooses to use can hurt, inspire, or do both at the same time.

I learned that people are much more complex than I might assume without digging, and that a deep conversation will many times reveal that the daily struggles of another are at least as difficult as my own.

I learned that being a patient, friend, father, and husband are roles that will be challenged by disease and suffering, but that, ultimately, it is the individual who has the power to define and accomplish his or her identity.

I learned that frustration and anger can be consuming, and that constant effort is necessary to triumph over them.

I learned that time and life move forward, regardless of whether things are happening according to plan, and that an acceptance of that fact can be freeing.

I learned that any shred of optimism is worth its weight in gold, regardless of whether or when it pans out.

I learned that people are defined much more accurately by how they overcome problems than by what those problems are to begin with.

I learned that some patients, like Jeff, are thrown into shocking physical illness; yet they retain the energy and grace to give selflessly of their time to help an unknown medical student learn to be a better doctor.

Time for Questions

DAVIS "MAC" STEPHEN

To divide fluid, human interactions into artificial categories reduces the capacity to represent lived experience, as it unfolds before us and as our emotions interpret each passing moment. However, the six months of knowing Mr. Sutton has compressed into my memory as three distinct categories: the doctor-patient interaction, the patient's outlook on experiencing illness, and a medical student's assessment of potential implications for being both a doctor and a patient.

My first meeting with Mr. Sutton was his appointment to decide on a plan for post-surgical chemotherapy—a decision that I envisioned would create an atmosphere of solemn, near-sacred gravity, since the treatment choice would likely determine his fate of life or death. I left his appointment feeling that I'd witnessed a busy yet experienced waitress give advice to a patron on the evening specials. This appointment, the second between Mr. Sutton and his oncologist, struck me as a remarkably rushed and routinized approach to deciding how one should battle cancer. Mr. Sutton had arrived—lawyerly—with yellow legal pad in hand, seemingly prepared to map-out options and weigh their relative merits. His oncologist, instead, delivered the oral *Spark* notes to explain chemotherapy for lung cancer. Mr. Sutton began receiving this information by scribbling down notes. He eventually put down the pen, as it could not keep pace with the logic or the vocabulary flooding towards him. Instead of returning home with his legal pad to research and consider the best choice for trying to save his life, he appeared to resolve, after being overwhelmed with science, that his oncologist's recommendation would do fine. "Yeah, I think we should go with that" were roughly his words of confirmation.

I've taken longer buying a set of golf clubs than Mr. Sutton took to decide his chemotherapy choice. This did not seem right to me. I've written these paragraphs to imply the same; however, I've reminded myself to be slower to judge. I'd been told by his oncologist that Mr. Sutton showed a tendency towards waffling about his medical decisions: what surgeon to see, whether to get a third opinion on chemotherapy, and so forth. Perhaps his oncologist chose to force a decision on Mr. Sutton to save crucial time from a medical perspective. Perhaps she presented the chemotherapy as such a standardized methodology to decrease his anxiety, seeking to imply that treatment courses are well-established and that what little mystery may exist isn't worth worrying over. Perhaps she never referred to the cancer as "his" to relieve any burden of ownership he may feel about the disease, or that the cancer was not something inherent to who he is.

While I remind myself that alternative interpretations of the doctor-patient interaction in this appointment are numerous, first impressions are hard to erase. The Mr. Sutton I still remember appeared nervous, frightened, and rapidly losing control over the fate of his own body and life. I hurt for him, to watch this man digest a 50-50 five-year survival prognosis and then find the wherewithal to make a confident, prompt decision about how to best fight the odds. Even if Mr. Sutton felt more confident than he appeared, he deserved the time to articulate that he felt so—or, really, to articulate anything.

As time later afforded, I found that Mr. Sutton's feelings about this appointment did reflect his appearance, or how I had interpreted it. During my first visit to his chemotherapy treatments, I asked how he felt about his oncologists' manner. He responded initially with forced praise, "Oh . . . she's great." Seeing that he wasn't sure what team I played for, I decided to shift away from purely open-ended tactics and just be honest with him. I let him know that I didn't know his oncologist well and that my allegiance was to him. I explained to him that I'd left their appointment feeling surprised by the expediency of the visit and decision, and I wondered if he felt the same way. He seemed to appreciate this confidentiality by admitting that he'd felt rushed and depersonalized, both from his cancer and its treatment decision. However, he remained positive about her manner, by saying he felt reassured that she'd insisted that he call her by her first name. Initially, this blew my mind. I should hope a patient would be on a first-name basis with the person who holds the keys to saving your life and/or caring for you while you die! However, as I would grow to know Mr. Sutton better, I would see this streak of optimism, generosity, and positive thinking return again and again. His fierce resilience against the many despairing realities he faced will be a topic I address in the next section, but it is a trend I first encountered in this moment.

Regardless of his oncologist's interpersonal manner, I also wanted to know how he felt about the treatment approach they had agreed on. He characterized his tendency towards indecision just as his oncologist had—that he'd received his cancer diagnosis at one hospital, sought a second-opinion from Dr. Montgomery, and still remained curious to know what the Cancer Center could have offered; however, he'd decided to stay with Dr. Montgomery for fear of losing valuable time. With this, I sensed a return of the nervous, uncertain Mr. Sutton that I'd seen in the first appointment. I gathered that, perhaps, this man places utmost priority on finding the most technically competent, medically-reliable physician possible, and less priority on a warm, pastor-like caregiver who understands what he's going through. To assuage his fears, I praised his oncologist's impressive training and research credentials, and reassured him that considering her line of research, few people on earth know more about the minutiae of his cancer and stay as up-to-date with best treatment practice as she does.

In my second visit to Mr. Sutton's chemotherapy session, he confirmed my suspicion of holding a competence-over-compassion rubric for evaluating physicians; yet, in the same visit, his girlfriend confirmed that the trait is not universal among patients. In the empty time we had to fill while Mr. Sutton sat receiving IV chemotherapy—bag after bag of, paradoxically, poisonous cure into his veins—I asked if he'd felt more invited to ask questions and discuss his treatment with Dr. Montgomery in their last visit. His girlfriend didn't give him time to respond. "What time for questions?" she asked me, with a smile animated by the anger she clearly still felt from the appointment. Without parsing her words, she explained that her father had lung cancer as well, and had received far more caring treatment than Mr. Sutton was receiving. She felt it was too late to change physicians, but nonetheless inexcusable for him to be treated as he had.

I noted that Mr. Sutton seemed bemused by her opinion. He agreed, perhaps out of appeasement to his raging girlfriend, that the "care" he receives is suboptimal. But he emphasized that competence is key to a physician's worth. He elaborated by saying he would rather have a "House MD" (referring to the grumpy but brilliant TV doctor) whose treatment decisions he can trust.

The structure of Mr. Sutton's analogy ("rather have House MD than . . .") implied to me that physicians often come in one variety or the other—competent or caring—but that the two qualities tend to mutually exclude one another. Patients' experiences in an over-worked, often underpaid, and definitely hectic US medical system probably lead to this conclusion quite often. TV programs and popular cultural conceptions—thanks in no small part to "House MD"—probably reinforce these patient experiences. What I've observed, as a first year medical student (with the added insight of a mother who teaches a mental health counseling graduate program), is that sound technique for conveying empathic support is not an extraordinary skill; rather, it requires a fairly human level of compassion for those suffering in plain sight, and a few standard questions to give patients the reins for sharing their feelings. Throughout this year interviewing patients for our patient-doctor course (PD1), and discussing the process with our preceptors, interpersonal "technique" seems potentially as simple as following a checklist. In fact, such checklists already exist thanks to one of our distinguished faculty, Dr. Arthur Kleinman, who patented the following "explanatory model" questions that a physician can ask a patient to evoke the patient's understanding and attitude towards his/her illness, regardless of cultural heritage:

- "What do you think has caused the illness?"
- "Why do you think it started when it did?"
- "What do you think your sickness does to you? How does it work?"
- "How severe is your sickness? Will it have a short course or long course?"
- "What kind of treatment do you think you should receive?"
- "What are the most important results you hope to receive from this treatment?"
- "What are the chief problems your sickness has caused for you?"
- "What do you fear most about your sickness?"

Especially because concern for others and the ability to memorize a few things are prerequisites for the medical field, my observations about this doctor-patient interaction led me to conclude that Mr. Sutton's representative "either-or attitude" about his physician's competence/compassion results less from poor social skills among our physicians (though we've all met *that* doctor who makes you wonder . . .) and more from the time available to our physicians. Mr. Sutton's oncologist certainly exemplified this distinction. Dr. Montgomery is a caring, compassionate physician. She immediately struck me as very self-aware and as willing to listen as talk.

However, in the appointments I joined, my private conversations with Mr. Sutton and his girlfriend, and private conversations with Dr. Montgomery, I saw little evidence that she had listened in a very meaningful way. In a lengthy packet of patient notes filled with relevant biological details of his illness, no reference is made to his explanatory model. The only vaguely related reference I can find is: "All questions answered, support provided." Even this weak assessment disagrees with my observations as well as his (and his girlfriend's) recounting of appointments. During my first visit to Mr. Sutton's chemotherapy session, I asked about his attitude towards this life-threatening disease he faced. He told me that his best friend, who eventually became his wife, had died of multiple sclerosis (MS) about a decade ago. Having functioned as her caregiver throughout the entirety of this illness, he viewed his lung cancer as far less severe. As easy as it was for me to evoke this personal anecdote of resilience from Mr. Sutton, I learned in my final visit with Dr. Montgomery that she did not know of his wife or her death, even after six months of being his oncologist. In this visit, I also asked what role, if any, she thought that the anxiety and excessive alcohol consumption may have played in his illness, because these issues were clearly listed in his past medical and social history. She said she had never addressed either of these issues.

While addressing a patient's explanatory model is strongly encouraged in our first-year patient-doctor course, discussing a patient's social history, alcohol use, and anxiety are among the building blocks of a first-year medical curriculum. How these features weren't being addressed in a premier cancer practice was, well, stunning.

Because I, like Mr. Sutton, felt faith in the competence of Dr. Montgomery, I pondered plausible explanations to my bewildering discovery. I reasoned that Dr. Montgomery practices up-to-date, evidenced-based medicine. As a practitioner and researcher, she is as current with literature on standard-of-care as anybody. She would not neglect any measures for emotionally supporting patients, if those measures were demonstrated to improve cure rates. Thus, addressing issues like Mr. Sutton's anxiety, possible alcohol abuse, and his own conception of his illness must be viewed by Dr. Montgomery as an amenity but not a necessity. Because of her pleasant personality, I also assumed she would enjoy relating to patients. Yet, because of her quick, efficient clinical demeanor, I was left to conclude that she simply lacks the time to address both medical and emotional needs. She would rather see one more patient, and possibly save one more life, than take an extra ten, maybe twenty minutes per patient, to delve into their psyche—simple as that.

I doubt I would have come to this beneficent conclusion had I known Dr. Montgomery did not address Mr. Sutton's emotional state during his treatment course. But now, with his surgery, chemotherapy, and cancer all behind him—medically a best-case scenario—I couldn't deny that she had done her job. She had reduced his cancer to nothing. Seeing this successful outcome and seeing the happiness Dr. Montgomery felt for Mr. Sutton, I realized that had Dr. Montgomery taken an extra ten or twenty minutes per patient to delve into complex social and emotional histories, she may not have had room on her panel for Mr. Sutton. For her, each irrelevant tangent during an interview begins adding up to another patient whom she won't have time to see, and, unlike Mr. Sutton, wouldn't have had time to cure.

This conclusion was initially troubling to me. I obviously didn't go to medical school to conclude that patients' subjective, tender, human sides slow physicians down. Luckily, at the end of this experience, I still don't settle with this conclusion. Instead, I feel thankful to have accompanied Mr. Sutton to a best-case outcome, while also realizing that things could have gone much, much worse. Had things gone worse—had the best-practice, evidence-based protocol failed—this man would have deserved for his caregiver to know him, understand him, and relate to him as he considered, approached, and faced death. Even if overwhelming evidence does not correlate explanatory models or empathy to superior outcomes, we, as physicians, owe our patients the dignity to walk what may be their final road side-by-side with them.

Fortunately, Dr. Montgomery did not have to walk this road with Mr. Sutton. Had his situation worsened, my experience showed that a physician—or even a lowly medical student like me—is granted special privilege into some of the closest, most personal aspects of a patient's life. Mr. Sutton, for example, shared with me one of his life's most painful experiences, and then related it to his outlook of a potentially terminal lung cancer. If such intense, special information can come to a student one-eighth of the way through medical school within thirty minutes of a visit, a physician with experience can probably elicit such a bond with patients in a matter of minutes. Recognizing when to take those minutes, and when those minutes may take away care from another patient, will be the art of medicine I forever strive to cultivate.

Eight Percent

MORGAN PRUST

Each year in early September, Rob's employer sponsors a blood drive in honor of a former employee, a passenger killed aboard one of the planes hijacked on September 11, 2001. Rob donated his blood every year, but this particular morning came in the middle of a special time. His son, Adam, was born two weeks earlier at the end of August, joining Rob, his wife Fran, and their two-and-a-half-year-old daughter, Lindsay, in their newly complete family. Beyond being the father of two young and active children, Rob was a computer programmer and personnel manager at a large and successful medical software company. At 36, he was living a happy life, and felt healthy as ever. So, when he was told that his blood count was too low to participate in the blood drive, Rob thought it was odd, but he didn't dwell on it.

Fall turned to winter, and that January, Massachusetts was pounded by almost weekly blizzards. Rob recalls coming in one Friday evening from a long session of snow-shoveling, feeling worn out and sore. He took some Advil and went to bed. The next morning, Rob got up to feed Lindsay breakfast. As he was sitting down with her at the table, he felt a sudden popping sensation on the left side of his abdomen, followed immediately by a warm rush of fluid. He realized he was sitting in a pool of blood, and ran for the bathroom near the kitchen, where he continued to bleed for about ten minutes. Much to his relief, the bleeding resolved on its own. He was shaken but felt fine, and his first thought was that he might have hemorrhoids. He cleaned himself up, took a shower, changed clothes, and took Lindsay to swim practice. By the time he got home, Fran was awake, and Rob told her what had happened. They agreed that he should see his physician as soon as possible, and scheduled an appointment for a colonoscopy, which allows the doctor to look inside the bowel for the source of bleeding.

Rob's father accompanied him to the colonoscopy appointment. After Rob had awoken from anesthesia, the doctor told Rob he encountered a stricture, an abnormal narrowing of the colon that prevented him from advancing the scope any further through the large intestine. Rob agreed to head into the hospital for some more tests. By the time he had been admitted it was early evening, and Rob told his dad to head home to get some rest. That night, he underwent an extensive battery of tests. He awoke the next morning to await the results.

As he sat on his bed waiting, a junior surgical resident came into his room. As she entered, she began to express her condolences, telling Rob how sorry she was about the news. Rob, not having spoken to any physicians that morning, and still in the dark about his test results, asked her to back up. "Wait, wait, wait," he interjected. He recalls that as she realized that Rob hadn't yet been given his diagnosis, a look of terror and mortification flashed on her face. "You mean, they haven't told you the results yet?" She told Rob that she would be right back with the attending surgeon who was on service that day, but Rob pressed her to tell him what was going on. She gave him a "barebones diagnosis," telling him that they had found what looked to be advanced Stage 4 colon cancer, but declined to give him any more detailed information before the attending surgeon had spoken with him. Once she left the room, Rob recalls feeling stunned, his mind reeling from what he had just heard. He decided to step outside for a breath of fresh air. On his cell phone, he typed "Stage 4 colon cancer" into a search query, and began to read the information that came up on the small screen—explaining that Stage 4 colon cancer means it has spread to other parts of the body. Rob thought, "Well, I'm going to die." As he sifted through websites on his phone, he read that 8 percent of patients survive Stage 4 colon cancer. At that moment, he said to himself, "I just have to be in that 8 percent."

Rob went back up to his room to find the surgical resident he had seen earlier, joined now by the attending physician. The doctor explained that Rob's scans had revealed a large mass in his colon, strongly suggestive of a cancer. The cancer appeared to have spread aggressively to the liver and lungs. As the physician described what they had seen on Rob's imaging studies, he explained that, while they would do everything they could, including surgical removal of the tumor in his colon followed by chemotherapy, it was unlikely that Rob had longer than a year to live.

He recalls only half-listening to what the doctor had to say. He listened to the doctor from a skeptical distance, the clumsiness of the delivery causing him to question everything he was hearing. Rob took everything in with a kind of defiance that allowed him to skip past feeling sad and sorry for himself. He wasn't going to break down. He was determined to get into the 8 percent.

As the dust settled, Rob was able to take stock of the situation, and began to prepare for what lay ahead. He called his wife, Fran, who left the children with a friend, and came up to Boston to join him. The physician who had come to see Rob that morning came back to explain the diagnosis to Fran. Rob recalls that she showed great strength as she took the news. She was embarking with him on a journey that would change their lives in fundamental ways. On the day that Rob received his diagnosis, he had to immediately prepare for the prospect of surgery. He stayed in the hospital over the weekend before the operation, during which time Fran traveled back and forth, switching off with Rob's parents to look after the kids in between trips up to Boston.

The next day, Rob went into the operating room. During the operation, the surgical team removed a foot-long section of

Rob's bowel, which included a "grapefruit-sized" mass. The cancer had invaded into the fatty tissue surrounding the colon and spread to the liver. Following the surgery, Rob stayed in the hospital for 10 days, and by the time he and Fran headed home, he hadn't seen Lindsay and Adam or slept in his own bed for two weeks. At this time, Rob was still planning to return to work as soon as possible, but remained unsure of what to expect in the weeks and months ahead, knowing that he would soon have to begin treatment with chemotherapy.

It was roughly two weeks later, in early March, when Rob and Fran had their first of what would be an ongoing series of meetings with Dr. Abrams throughout that spring, summer, and fall. As Rob's medical oncologist, he would be overseeing the administration of chemotherapy in the months to come. As they sat down for their first meeting, they agreed that given Rob's young age, that he was otherwise strong and healthy, and that he was the father of two young children, it made sense to be as aggressive as possible in their approach to therapy. As he had felt since the day he received his diagnosis the previous month, Rob was determined to try everything and endure anything, not wanting to look back in regret for not having done more. He knew the odds he was up against, and Dr. Abrams made it clear that there was no way to know what outcomes to expect from the chemotherapy, but they decided to try as hard as they could and hope for a positive response.

Rob and Fran started making the trip to the hospital every two weeks. Rob would check into the lab for blood testing, meet for a consultation with Dr. Abrams to discuss any clinical issues that Rob was experiencing, and then proceed down the hall to sit for his infusion. The chemotherapy pods are spacious, semi-private bays with large windows overlooking the hospital parking lot and the greenery beyond it. Rob and Fran came to know this space very intimately, and over Rob's six months of treatment, he never stopped hating this biweekly ritual, but gradually settled into a routine.

As with all chemotherapy, there were side effects. When I ask Rob to describe his experience of chemotherapy, the predominant sensation he recalls is intense and persistent nausea, akin to the feeling of having drunk too much alcohol, without the relief that usually accompanies throwing up. As I listened to Rob describe this feeling, I thought of "A Queasy Feeling," Atul Gawande's chapter on nausea, from his book *Complications*. He describes nausea as a "strange and awful beast," one that is much more aversive and deeply felt than pain. "Break a leg on a ski slope," he writes, "and—as bad as traumatic pain can be—once you can, you'll ski again. After one unfortunate experience with a bottle of gin or an oyster, by contrast, people won't go near the culprit for years." Nausea was clearly a defining feature of Rob's experience with chemotherapy, and, as he and Fran describe it, his infusion cycles followed a fairly regular two-week pattern. For the first three days after his Wednesday infusion, Rob would be more or less bedridden, intensely nauseous, and completely exhausted. While he was able to get modest relief from his nausea with medications, he simply felt too ill and depleted to do anything but sleep, unable even to read in bed. By Saturday morning, he was usually able to reemerge from bed, and the following 10 days leading up to the next infusion were a gradual process of recovering and gaining strength for the next round of treatment. Rob endured 14 chemotherapy treatments. While Rob doesn't discount the brutal challenges he endured during this time, he talks about it without melodrama, and recalls that he did his best to keep life as normal as possible. On the days he was not confined to his bed, he and Fran enjoyed getting out of the house to take day trips with Lindsay and Adam. Rob had always enjoyed exercising, but now approached fitness with a new level of seriousness, viewing it as a core part of the healing process, and running up to five miles each day on his basement treadmill.

Rob got his first piece of positive feedback for all his hard work in early May, when a scan revealed that the liver lesions had either shrunk dramatically or shown no signs of significant growth. This was clearly good news, and, at their meeting with Dr. Abrams, they began to consider the possibility of surgery to remove Rob's liver lesions. Dr. Abrams arranged for Rob and Fran to have their first of many meetings with Dr. Corbett, the liver surgeon. The meeting lasted over an hour, during which time they discussed the pros and cons of removing the cancer in the liver. They also discussed Rob's surprisingly positive response to chemotherapy, as seen on his latest scan. In the end, they reached the conclusion that, unfortunately, Rob was not a candidate for liver resection at that time. Dr. Corbett did say, however, that it was reasonable to continue his chemotherapy and reevaluate the possibility of liver resection in a few months.

Rob and Fran have nothing but respect and admiration for Dr. Corbett (and, indeed, Lindsay is fond of parading around their living room in the character of "Dr. Corbett-the-super-hero"), but they were disappointed after this meeting. They had become excited by the prospect of a potentially cancer-eliminating surgery, but Rob pressed on with his treatments and was more than happy to be done.

A repeat scan showed that his efforts had continued to pay off, with significant further shrinkage of his liver metastases. Rob recounts that, when they met with Dr. Corbett again in to review his scans and revisit the possibility of liver resection, Dr. Corbett "wasn't doing backflips;" but, in light of Rob's age and two young children, he was willing to take a holistic view of the risks and rewards of surgery. While Rob's scan showed an excellent response to therapy, he still was not an ideal candidate for liver surgery. Given Rob's life circumstances, however, Dr. Corbett was willing to keep the door open. Rob understood that most patients with liver resection experience a recurrence, and while the probabilities were not high, the operation offered a chance of cure. After months of waiting, Rob and Fran had no doubt this was their preferred course of action.

On the day of Rob's surgery, I walked over to the hospital. I was greeted by Kara, the third-year medical student rotating with Dr. Corbett that month on her surgical clerkship. We had a few minutes to chat before Dr. Corbett joined us, and I had a thousand questions, which Kara very patiently answered for me. After Dr. Corbett came to meet us, he took me to see Rob and Fran. They were in a bay of the pre-surgical unit, Rob lying in a hospital bed and Fran sitting next to him. Dr. Corbett told them that I was the medical student that he'd told them about, and that I would be following Rob's case for the next few months. They were very warm and welcoming, and the conversation quickly turned to the sequence of events that would unfold over the course of the day. Dr. Corbett explained the procedure to them, and told them that it would take roughly six hours, after which Rob would be brought out of anesthesia and taken to the recovery room before moving up to the inpatient ward. Fran jokingly asked Dr. Corbett if he'd had his coffee that morning. After a few more laughs, a look of sincerity returned to Dr. Corbett's face, and, as we left, he looked at Fran and said "We're going to take good care of him."

Dr. Corbett led me through a snaking maze of hallways, elevators, and double doors, and, after changing out of my clothes into surgical scrubs, I met Kara by the sink, where she showed me how to scrub my hands, meticulously getting under the finger nails and into all the little nooks between the fingers, where bacteria might like to hide. Hands and forearms clean, we went into the operating room, where the team of surgical residents, anesthesiologists, and nurses were all getting ready. Jesse, a very talkative scrub nurse, helped me on with my gloves, surgical gown, and eye shield. Dr. Corbett introduced me to Luke, the chief resident in surgery who would be assisting with the operation, as well as the other nurses who would be working in the OR. Soon, everyone assumed his or her place around the operating table, where Rob lay with the sterile drapes around him. Dr. Corbett and Luke stood on either side of Rob's abdomen. Jesse, the scrub nurse, stood next to Dr. Corbett by the table of operating instruments, a vast and completely sterile array of clamps, scissors and sutures. On the other side of the table, Kara stood next to Luke and I stood next to Kara, by Rob's right foot.

Dr. Corbett explained the procedure to me as he proceeded. He made a large incision to expose the abdominal cavity, which was held open by metal retractors for the duration of the operation. At one point, Dr. Corbett invited me to feel one of the liver tumors. I placed my gloved fingers on the liver, and felt Rob's heart beating through his diaphragm. It was a moment I won't ever forget. I felt the awesome force with which medicine and illness thrust people into each other's lives.

About halfway through the surgery, once the right lobe was removed, Dr. Corbett asked one of the nurses to call up to the waiting area to let Fran know that everything was going well, and that it would be a few more hours until they were finished. Fran had remarked to me a few times how meaningful this small gesture was for her, and that, while it helped her not to worry too much as she paced back and forth in the waiting room, it also showed how much Dr. Corbett cared, not just about Rob but about her as well. The operation proceeded without complication. I was absolutely awestruck for its entire duration.

In our medical school curriculum, we had just finished our eight-week block of human anatomy. Three or four days each week that fall, we spent our mornings in the dissection lab with our cadavers, wielding scalpels and scissors in the service of getting to know how the human body is put together in all its striking complexity. But dissecting a cadaver is a learning exercise on a body that is cold and grey and fixed with formaldehyde. In surgery, the tissues are brightly colorful, warm, and pulsing with life. The tissues behave according to the unforgiving laws of human physiology, and exposed under the lights, can be seen serving their life-sustaining purposes. As I witnessed Rob's surgical team manipulate the phenomenally complex task of excising the diseased segments of Rob's liver, I had trouble getting over how miraculous it all was.

After roughly six-and-a-half hours, the operation was complete, and all the tissue margins had been confirmed by a pathologist to be negative for tumor tissue. The incision was carefully closed, every suture and surgical instrument was painstakingly accounted for, and Rob was slowly brought out of anesthesia. By the end of the operation, I realized how sore my shoulders and legs were, though it was a small price to pay for the chance to witness this component of Rob's treatment.

After taking off my gloves and gown, I accompanied Dr. Corbett and Kara to talk to Fran. We found her in the waiting area, and we all sat down in a small consultation room. Fran shed tears of joy and gratitude, giving Dr. Corbett a hug when he told her that the operation had been a success. As Dr. Corbett described everything that surgical team had done over the course of the afternoon, Fran got out her notepad to take down the information. "I'm so happy, I'm never going to remember all these details," she said. Dr. Corbett replied, "All you need to remember is that he did great, and that I couldn't be happier with how things went."

As Rob recovered from surgery, I visited him regularly over his nine days of inpatient recovery. Over the first few days, Rob was naturally exhausted, and during my visits, I would sit and talk with Fran while he slept. As his liver recovered from the trauma it had just endured, Rob experienced some fluid build-up, as well as the abdominal pain and fatigue that necessarily accompany an operation like his. During his nine-day inpatient stay, Fran would drive up to Boston each morning, leaving the kids with her parents. While this was by no means a pleasant time for Rob, he made a steady and un-complicated recovery; and, as I visited him over those nine days, I was impressed by how much color and energy he gained between each visit. On the third day after surgery, I came into his room to find him sitting upright in a chair, show-ing little sign of the challenge he faced.

Early on in my relationship with Rob, I think I struggled with the ambiguity of my role. I could not help feeling like an intruder, an unwanted witness to Rob's illness, with nothing to offer but my interest in his and Fran's experience of illness. From my own experience as a surgical patient, I knew how ex-hausting it is to have visitors in the hospital after a major oper-ation, and I worried that Rob and Fran would see me as little more than a burdensome nuisance. I did my best not to let my self-consciousness show, but I'm not sure I was always suc-cessful. Nonetheless, Rob and Fran were extremely generous in sharing their time and energy with me, helping me understand the story of Rob's illness as it had unfolded over the previous year.

As Rob and Fran shared the challenges they had confront-ed in living with Rob's diagnosis, they deepened my under-standing of what it is to live with cancer, both in terms of Rob's bodily experience of his illness and how its effects had played out in their lives as a young family. While they had been in the fortunate financial position of being able to put their careers on hold, they were not relieved of the full-time job of being parents to a 1-year-old and a 3-year-old, whose pictures were on the windowsill of Rob's hospital room.

They also told me that while Rob's illness had helped strengthen their relationship with Fran's parents, who were happy to play a more active role as grandparents and caretakers to Lindsay and Adam, it had complicated their relations with Rob's extended family. As Rob later explained to me, during his first hospitalization in February, misunderstandings between Fran and Rob's parents, regarding who would be making decisions on Rob's behalf, boiled over into tensions that remain complicated even now. These complexities were further exacerbated by the need for genetic screening of each of Rob's immediate family members. At the suggestion of Rob's medical team, each of his siblings and parents were screened for genetic risk for the known causes of hereditary colorectal cancer. Each of Rob's immediate relatives tested negative for the genetic risk of these conditions, although, with oddly coincidental timing, his mother was also diagnosed with colon cancer.

Over the course of his nine inpatient days and clinic visits throughout the winter and early spring, we kept our conversation going week by week. Many of my most memorable moments with Rob and Fran took place before and after our meetings with Dr. Corbett and Dr. Abrams. I met Rob and Fran in the lobby of the hospital. It was the first time I had seen them since Rob was discharged from the hospital, and Rob joked that this was the first time I had ever seen him standing up. We went upstairs to the oncology office, and, as we sat in the waiting room before seeing Dr. Corbett and Dr. Abrams, Rob and Fran told me the story of how they met during Rob's summer as Fran's intern.

During the consultation that afternoon, we discussed the next phase of Rob's treatment. He had had another round of imaging that morning, and his scans indicated that he remained cancer-free; but, as part of the treatment protocol, he was preparing for another round of chemotherapy. This so-called "mop up" chemotherapy was intended to target any latent tumor cells not visible on diagnostic imaging. Unlike his first experience with chemotherapy, this round would involve only four to six cycles, if his scans continued to look good at the end of it. In order to commence this next round of treatments, however, Rob needed to have recovered sufficiently from his surgery, and Dr. Corbett was concerned about his weight. Rob looked drawn and thin, and Fran was put in charge of making sure that Rob took in enough calories to be able to withstand his therapies.

Two weeks later, Rob's weight had rebounded, coming back up by five or six pounds, and he was declared ready to start his next phase of chemotherapy. I joined him and Fran and, as we waited to see Dr. Abrams' nurse before Rob's infusion, Fran commented on how strange it felt being back at the hospital. It had been four months since Rob finished his first round of chemotherapy, and being back there naturally brought back intense memories, as though they were returning to the scene of a crime.

We sat down for a quick meeting with the nurse, who went over Rob's recent health history from his post-operative recovery period, and performed a physical exam. Rob, understandably wary of having to go through any more chemotherapy than he absolutely had to, asked how many rounds of treatment he would have to do, noting that there had been some ambiguity over whether it would be four or six. The nurse replied that Dr. Abrams had decided to give him six rounds of treatment, because they wanted to do everything they could to get Rob into the percentage of patients who survive Stage 4 disease. With that, we walked down the hall to the infusion pods. Rob and Fran greeted the nurses and social workers like old friends, and, as Rob got situated in his chair, his nurse began the infusions through the port in Rob's chest. I sat with Fran and Rob through the beginning of the infusion, with Rob stoically tolerating his reunion with his much-hated medications, and gradually succeeding in drifting off to sleep. As I left them to head back to school for my afternoon classes, we made a plan to see each other two weeks later for the next infusion;

and Fran and I agreed to be in touch over the next couple of days, for an update on how Rob was tolerating his medications.

That first cycle of his mop-up treatments would be the hardest of all the chemotherapy that Rob endured by the end of his treatment. He began experiencing a sharp, constant stabbing pain in his lower abdomen over the weekend following his infusion. It lasted for an entire week, not responding to any pain medications, but, as mysteriously as it had arrived, it disappeared the following weekend. But debilitating as this pain was, it didn't stop Rob and Fran from marking the one-year anniversary of Rob's diagnosis. Instead of watching the Super Bowl in a hospital room, they were at home; and, contrary to the physician's prediction on the day of Rob's diagnosis, he was alive and by all indications, cancer-free.

Rob's treatments proceeded more or less without complication, and, as he endured the cyclical routine, he found ways of keeping himself busy. He joined a fitness program at his local YMCA, geared specifically toward cancer patients undergoing chemotherapy. Rob liked to joke that he was about 30 years younger than the next oldest person in his class, and that, as a result, he could run laps around them. Just as he had during his first round of treatments, Rob did his best to keep things normal, making the most of the days he was able to be active and out of bed, and keeping his sights set on the end of treatment.

In mid-March, I was away from Boston for a week of spring vacation, and called Rob on the phone to check in with how he was doing. He said that in general he was feeling fine, but that, in the past week or so, he had begun to have an uncomfortable sensation of tightness in the region around his liver. It wasn't painful exactly, but it felt like someone was squeezing his liver. On the other hand, he was feeling happy because Dr. Abrams had decided to scale his treatments down to four cycles. Rob's next and final infusion was scheduled for Wednesday of the following week, after which he would wait two weeks before coming back to Boston for another set of scans.

Though I knew how important it was to manage my own expectations, I couldn't help but feel a certain hopeful anticipation, as I walked through the front door of the hospital. It was a clear, sunny day, and the weather was pleasantly, if unseasonably, warm. Today, there would be no chemotherapy or infusions. Rob had arrived earlier that morning for a round of diagnostic imaging: an MRI and CT scan. His chemotherapy complete, it was a big day, and it felt like a moment of truth.

When I met Rob and Fran in the waiting room, I found them more excited than anxious. Rob had managed to keep on all of his weight, and his time at the gym left him feeling and looking healthy. His skin had good color, and the soreness around his surgical incision had abated to the point that he could pick up his one-year-old son again. The tightness in his abdomen persisted, but other than that he was feeling good. Fran remarked that it was 14 months to the day since they had received his diagnosis. Holding Rob's hand, she smiled and said, "Today feels like graduation day."

I knew that the natural history of metastatic colon cancer made it too soon to breathe a sigh of relief, but it was hard not to feel caught up with them in this moment they had been waiting for over so many months. After two major surgeries and 18 grueling cycles of chemotherapy, they were more than ready to settle into the slower rhythms of life after treatment. After a few more weeks of letting Rob recover from his last cycle, they were planning to pack up the car and take the kids on a road trip, either to Hershey Park in Pennsylvania, or, even more boldly, to Disney World. "We're just going to get in the car and go," Fran said.

And so it was with nervous hope that I sat with Rob and Fran that afternoon in early April, waiting for Dr. Abrams to report the long-anticipated imaging results, and chatting about their plans to take to the open road. The nurse working at front desk signaled to us that we could go into the exam room, and that Dr. Abrams would be with us shortly. No sooner had we sat down than Dr. Abrams entered the room. He shook hands with Rob, Fran, and me, and, as we all sat down, he launched into the news.

"Well, your scan is showing a number of complexities," he said, "some of them not so worrying but others a little more worrying." The positive energy drained out of the room as quickly as Dr. Abrams had entered it, and for a painful five seconds, nobody said anything. Dr. Abrams went on to explain that Rob's scans showed a large fluid collection in the liver. There was a new lung nodule that had not been present on the previous scan. Most worryingly, the studies suggested the possibility that Rob's colon had formed an abnormal connection, known as a fistula, with his healing liver tissue, putting him at significant risk for bacterial contamination of his bloodstream. It was only after this long list of troubling results that he mentioned that Rob's liver showed no signs of recurrent cancer. When Dr. Abrams had got through delivering the news from the radiologist's report, Rob asked, "So what do we need to do now?" Dr. Abrams said that another surgical procedure was probably going to be necessary, but did not want to be specific about what that might be before talking to Dr. Corbett. Fran was struggling to write everything down in her notebook, asking clarifying questions like "What do you mean by 'a fistula'?"

As the meeting progressed, I was surprised by Dr. Abrams's use of medical jargon, and how much confusion could have been avoided by simply discussing Rob's imaging findings in lay terms. If part of being an effective clinician is being a skilled translator, I felt that Dr. Abrams was not making it easy to understand the news. Beyond the linguistic disconnect, big questions hung in the air. If there was a fistula, why wasn't Rob sick? If he had to have another surgery, what options would be on the table? Were the lung nodules something to worry about, or, like Rob's earlier lung nodules, would they recede? After more back and forth, Fran's disappointment and frustration came to a head, and, trying to stay calm and hold back her tears, she said, "I feel like there's something you're not telling us, Dr. Abrams! I wish you would just be straight with us!"

Dr. Abrams walked us through the radiologist's report again, emphasizing more vehemently the lack of cancer in the liver, and, while several major questions lingered, Dr. Abrams would arrange for a meeting with Dr. Corbett as soon as possible, to discuss the surgical management of Rob's imaging results. As the meeting was wrapping up and we were getting ready to leave, Rob, with his unflappable decency, placed his hand on Dr. Abrams' desk, and, looking him in the eye, said, "I really appreciate all you've done for me."

Walking out of the clinic toward the elevators, Rob said, "I had a feeling it was going to be something like this. My liver hasn't felt right for the last few weeks." In tears, Fran said, "I just want this to be over; I can't keep doing this; I'm totally exhausted." Empathizing with their disappointment, and trying for the moment to keep my own in check, I told them to keep in mind the bottom line that Rob's liver remained cancer-free, and that, while Dr. Abrams had sketched out a gloomy scenario about the possibility of a fistula, for the moment there was no evidence at all that Rob was sick. They asked me to translate some of the complex vocabulary from the meeting, and, though it was painful and sorely disappointing moment for everyone present, I was happy to be able to help them with the aftermath of the meeting, in the small ways that I could.

After two anxious days of waiting, the three of us met with Dr. Corbett that Friday. He explained that, while the radiologist no doubt had the best of intentions, they had never seen or examined Rob personally, so their diagnostic reading was out of touch with the reality of Rob's case. If Rob had had a fistula between his colon and his liver, Dr. Corbett explained, he would have developed a serious infection and all of the systemic symptoms associated with it. He believed that the large fluid collection in the liver was likely bile, and that the fluid would need to be drained, but that this could be done in a relatively straightforward, outpatient procedure. After the fluid was removed, they would leave a drain in temporarily, and then, ultimately, place a more permanent internal tube, or "stent," inside the bile ducts, in order to decrease leakage into the liver. Finally, he believed it was too early to know whether the lung nodules were of any significance, and that we would have to simply wait to see how they behaved over time.

This meeting transformed the outlook for Rob's treatment substantially. While he would need a series of further procedures over the coming weeks, which would require more trips to Boston and force them to place their road trip on hold, it was a tremendous relief to no longer be facing a third open-abdominal surgery and the months of recovery that it would entail. Rob came back up to Boston the following Wednesday to have his liver drained, and the fluid was, indeed, bile. They removed a large amount of fluid, the exact volume of a bottle of wine, he jokingly reported to me afterward; and the sense of relief he felt in his abdomen was immediate. He no longer had the feeling of tightness and fullness in his right-upper quadrant, and felt that a great pressure was relieved, much to his satisfaction.

Over the following two weeks, Rob learned to tolerate life with a drain in his abdomen. In addition to feeling odd and vaguely uncomfortable, it required him to wrap himself in plastic wrap before taking a shower. His fluid outputs remained consistently high in the days after his draining procedure, and, after two weeks of waiting for them to come down, Dr. Corbett decided that it was time for Rob to have an internal drain or stent placed, so the fluid would drain into his intestines. The procedure was conducted under general anesthesia and took about an hour. When he woke up, he reported feeling a sharp pain in his abdomen, but, other than that, he was feeling fine. The pain gradually subsided over the next couple of days, but was made a bit worse after he stopped for doughnuts on the way home.

While the end of Rob's chemotherapy failed to usher in the much hoped-for end of his active treatment, it is amazing to reflect on where he is and how he is doing today, relative to the likely outcomes that were spelled out for him at the time of diagnosis. He is not only alive but healthy, active, and eager to get back to work. His treatment and clinical course seem to have shifted into a new phase over the past two months. Last year, his cancer treatments were a fulltime job that his and Fran's lives were centered around, each and every day. They can both recall instantly and effortlessly the date of every appointment, every procedure, and every decision that was made along their forced march through the worlds of cancer treatment.

More and more, however, it seems like they have regained the freedom to think about other things. Instead of day trips to Boston, they are planning road trips to places like Pennsylvania, North Carolina, and Florida. Rob and Fran happily debate when Rob should go back to work. They are even thinking of moving to be closer to Rob's place of work, in a school district they like better.

Rob and Fran have been affected deeply by what they've come through, and they know that their journey is not over. Rob will require careful observation with regular colonoscopies and CT scans for the foreseeable future. It is impossible to eliminate the risk of recurrence, and that awareness is something they will always carry with them. Rob's young age at diagnosis also means that Lindsay and Adam will need to be carefully monitored for colon cancer throughout their lives, with regular screening procedures starting at age 25 for each of them. As Siddhartha Mukherjee observes in *The Emperor of*

All Maladies, the word "oncology" derives from "*onkos*"—Greek for mass or burden. Rob has fared extraordinarily well for a patient with his diagnosis, not because his burden had been light, but because he has marched forward with strength and determination, despite its heaviness. And, indeed, he hasn't marched alone. Who could?

While I wasn't there, I heard that when Rob and Fran brought Lindsay and Adam up to Boston for a meeting with Dr. Corbett last year, Lindsay said to him, "Thank you for saving my daddy's life." When I met Dr. Corbett for the first time last fall, he told me that surgical oncology involves a large dose of psychiatry, and that, beyond being skilled in the intricacies of surgical technique, being a good surgical oncologist means being emotionally present with each patient and committed to the long arc of their care. Following Dr. Corbett in the clinic and observing him, it is clear how attentively he listens to each of his patients, and that each of them feels how deeply he cares about his role in their treatment. The combination of skill and empathy he has brought to Rob's care are no doubt central to how well Rob is doing today.

Fran's commitment to Rob's successful treatment and recovery is awe-inspiring, as indispensible as any medication or surgery. I have never seen Rob without Fran at his side. Always ready with her pen and well-worn notebook during clinic appointments, she could easily teach a course at Harvard Medical School. Despite all of the fear and hardship she has overcome in the past 16 months, her good humor, warmth, and kindness appear unchanged by this ordeal. The solidarity that defines Rob and Fran's relationship is something that I will always remember in my future career, as I care for patients, and in my own life. They are testament to the truth that, while we cannot shoulder heavy burdens alone, extraordinary weight can be carried, and amazing things achieved, through the forces of love and human connection.

Reflections on a Journey

EUGENE VAIOS

A glass wall separated me from the patient that I was to follow for the next few months of my first year in medical school. When I received my assignment, I was ecstatic. A seasoned burn surgeon, Army corporal, and one of Harvard's finest mentors would be taking me under his wing, and introducing me to the world of healing, listening, and understanding the patients I would one day have the privilege to serve. But as I stood behind that glass wall, I wondered if I was ready for Andriy, and prepared to cross the divide between us. Would I have the strength to hide the pain in my heart and the tears welling up behind my eyes? As I watched the scene unfolding, my legs rooted to the ground and my eyes fixed, nurses were removing bandages from the writhing body of an almost unrecognizable 8-year-old boy. His only fault in life was having been at the wrong place at the wrong time.

Andriy was born in a rural town on the outskirts of Ukraine. He had never been to America, had no intention to visit, and probably had never even heard of the United States. As the picture hanging in his hospital room suggests, he had been a handsome young boy, with silky blonde hair and a love for soccer. But all of that changed. According to Dr. Grove, the accident happened in a barn. Everyone except Andriy had escaped, unharmed. The events that transpired that day were unclear, but, over the next few weeks, the puzzle pieces would slowly come together, and I would learn what brought an innocent boy nearly 5,500 miles away from home.

It had been a week since Dr. Grove and I met for the first time at the burn hospital. Though located in the heart of Boston, its physicians care for patients from all corners of the globe. I was anxious to finally meet Andriy. The last time I arrived at the hospital, he was still in the intensive care unit

(ICU), and nurses were replacing bandages from a recent surgery. I remember his legs kicking and arms flailing, as the staff repeatedly tried to console Andriy with soothing words of encouragement and promises that the pain would soon be over. I had stared, transfixed, at the bandaged body in front of me. He was covered in white bandages, with only his face untouched. Beneath all the cables, tubes, and anguish was a child who longed for his family, normalcy, and the innocence he had once known. I had watched the scene unfold until one of the nurses pulled the curtain around the bed closed, and Dr. Grove nudged me away from the glass wall where I stood.

Now, as I looked into the ICU room, Andriy was nowhere to be seen. The window curtains were pulled, the bed was empty, the nurses were gone, and the beeping machines were silent. It was a Saturday afternoon and the floor was unusually quiet. It was 10 a.m. on a cold, November morning: The wind and signs of cold were visible from between the curtains of the room. I wondered how many times he had looked out that window, while trapped in his sterile bubble, searching between the towering skyscrapers of the Boston skyline for a sign of his distant home. As I looked on, I squeezed the faded, black, leather notebook in my palm, in which I had scribbled several questions while sitting anxiously in the lobby. In reality, my questions had little chance of being answered. I would have to discover new ways to communicate with my patient, ways that could cross the language barrier that separated us. Indeed, Andriy's last few months had been a journey. And I, too, was about to embark on a journey of my own.

I turned from the empty room and looked down the corridor for the nurse who had greeted me on my way in. Standing in front of the nursing desk was Dr. Piedmont, a burn surgeon and colleague of Dr. Grove's. We had first met in my HMS anatomy course. Dr. Piedmont stood out in my memory for his heartwarming smile and jovial personality. For the children who came for burn treatment, he must have been a beacon of hope. I introduced myself and asked if he knew anything about Andriy's whereabouts. According to Dr. Piedmont, he had been moved out of the ICU to the seventh floor. As Dr. Piedmont led me toward the stairwell, I followed close at his heels, eager for what awaited us below. As we wound our way down the flight of stairs, he recounted Andriy's journey.

Andriy arrived with nearly 80 percent of his skin burned off. As I would soon find out, the digits on his hands were also burned off, leaving behind small stubs. His face was spared, but his ears were unrecognizable. In an effort to cover his burns with intact skin from elsewhere on his body, the Ukrainian surgeons took skin from his scalp. His body was frail and drained of its energy after a long battle for survival. His wounds were infected with drug-resistant bacteria, forcing the hospital to use a toxic drug that could defeat the disease but also risked harming the patient. Managing burn patients is no easy task, and, as Andriy would learn, the road to recovery is not only challenging but also long. Post-traumatic stress disorder is reported in one-third of burn survivors. Contracture and hypertrophy of scars must also be addressed immediately, to minimize deformity and optimize rehabilitation. As I processed all of this, I admired the mural on the staircase wall. It was a colorful scene from the tropics, rich with foreign animals and imagery of a happier time. The artist who painted the mural wanted it to be an escape from suffering, not only for the patients but also for the physicians.

Dr. Piedmont introduced me to the nurses and directed me to Andriy's room. I crossed the threshold and entered. The room was large and empty except for Andriy, who lay in his bed, and the tall, thin woman who stood protectively beside him. As we entered the room, she looked up from Andriy and greeted us with a warm smile, her radiant blue eyes injecting the room with a sense of hope and calm. Her fair skin and long, blond hair betrayed her Ukrainian roots. She reminded me of an exotic bird that was lost, one that would have been at home in the tropical mural, but was instead trapped inside the cage of our complex health care system, from which there seemed no escape. And yet, somehow, she managed to muster that smile and continue pretending that everything that was happening in her life was normal, that everything was going to be okay.

As Aleksandra redirected her attention to Andriy, Dr. Piedmont and I stood on the other side of the bed, while he updated me on Andriy's health. He was being treated with antibiotics to combat his infections. The burns on his arms were covered with negative pressure bandages to promote skin healing. Beneath his purple pajama pants and red A.S. Roma shirt, his body was noticeably frail, after months of struggle. His face was spared, but the rest of his head was covered in bandages. Over the last 5 months, he endured over 40 operations and, on several occasions, nearly died from sepsis. The smiling boy waving back at me was a living miracle.

Andriy seemed attentive and, after Dr. Piedmont's kind reintroduction to Andriy's aunt, quickly returned his gaze to the cartoons on the television across his bed. After checking in with Aleksandra, Dr. Piedmont turned to me, wished me well, and left the room in a flash. When Dr. Piedmont's heel disappeared around the corner of the door, I was left alone with Aleksandra, Andriy, and the beeping machines. Here I was, dressed in a tie and my white coat, eager to ask many questions, but unsure where to begin. As I looked around the room, I noticed the unopened containers of fruit and yogurt that sat on the table to his right. According to Aleksandra, he was drinking apple juice and eating some foods, but had minimal appetite for the American cuisine. Sandwiches and burgers were an inadequate substitute for the smell and taste of home-cooked Ukrainian cuisine. I noticed he had a tracheostomy and a feeding tube, scars from his past battles, which Dr. Piedmont promised would soon be removed. Aleksandra explained that he was learning to use the bathroom on his own, but needed her assistance to walk from his bed. Despite all the doctors and nurses, she played an active role in his care. She could not have been more than 30 years old. Yet, as she played with the bandages on his left arm and lovingly fixed his shirt, it was obvious that she was more than just an aunt; she was a mother, a friend, a caretaker, and a symbol of hope. One could sense her immense love for the boy who stared ahead at the television screen across from his bed, seemingly oblivious of the new stranger who had entered his life.

As I absorbed the scene, I noticed the treasure of toys, such as stuffed animals, action figures, trucks, balloons, and blow-up characters, which lined his window. It was an impressive collection for a child who had been in America for only 5 months, a collection equivalent to what many children would consider a lifetime of Christmas holidays. I wondered where the gifts had come from, how many people had passed through his life, what the gifts meant to him, and whether there was a gift he still longed for—a gift that, maybe, could not be bought in a toy store. Given his 40 operations, these treasures were probably milestones marking all the turns in his miraculous journey. Andriy deserved a room full of presents, I said to myself. Aleksandra broke my thoughts and pointed to the prize of them all, which sat at the foot of the bed. Arek was a giant, blue sea turtle. He was a replacement for Andriy's stuffed animal from Ukraine, which had been lost in the hospital during his first few days in America. The toy was never found, and Aleksandra shared that Andriy cried for days. As I processed her words, I wondered how much loss he had endured during his short life. His blue, innocent eyes seemed tired and aged. What looked like a frail boy was actually a grown man who had seen, suffered, and endured. Like his stuffed animal, he, too, was lost in

289

a foreign world and in a complex, fragmented medical system. Unlike the stuffed animal, however, he is irreplaceable. The love with which Aleksandra massaged his bandages told me why she, too, had traveled halfway across the world for him, and that no sea turtle, picture, or memory could replace this young boy full of promise. She was determined to bring him home.

Courtney, the physical therapist, entered the room for his 10 a.m. exercise routine. Trailing behind her was Lisa, another staff member and former burn patient. Courtney's contagious energy and enthusiasm exploded into the room and nearly lifted Andriy from his bed. Lisa was also talkative and had a bubbly personality. Their first task for the day was walking around the hospital floor. Aleksandra gathered his cables and the negative pressure-machine connected to his bandages. Meanwhile, Andriy struggled to prop himself up on his elbows and shift his body to the edge of the bed. Completely unaided, he slowly slid off the bed. As he struggled to gain his balance, his body swayed like a house propped on sticks in the middle of a hurricane. His legs shook and his arms shot out to his sides to steady himself. Aleksandra, the nurses, and I readied ourselves to catch his fall, but somehow he managed without us. Each step seemed like a mile, but, in a few minutes, the five of us were out the door and in the hallway.

As we walked around the floor, Lisa admitted how remarkable it was to see Andriy alive and walking. She shared that during his first few months in the hospital, the staff were not sure if he would make it. Yet, here he was, living, breathing, and making progress with every step. Courtney was standing by his side, holding him by the waist for support, while Aleksandra walked backwards in front of him, occasionally speaking to him in Russian and translating for the rest of us in broken English. At each turn in the hallway, Lisa told Andriy to stop and take a deep breath. His breaths were labored, as if every muscle in his body was being called upon to expand his chest. Eventually, Courtney told Andriy to try walking without her help. She removed her hands and gave him an encouraging smile. Aleksandra beckoned him to keep going, but Andriy stood there, rooted to the ground. Time stood still as we looked on. And then it happened. The boy who just moments ago seemed unfazed finally cracked. Our Superman was human.

The tears fell like rain down his cheeks, his shoulders shuddering and his chest heaving like waves in the middle of a storm. Reality finally caught up with Andriy. His energy was spent. Watching the scene unfold, I felt a tug at my heart. I too wanted to cry. I wanted to cry for Andriy and for the countless other patients around us who had been at the wrong place at the wrong time, and whose childhoods had been stolen from under their feet. He was only 8 years old, and yet he had endured more than some experience in a lifetime. In this moment, Andriy was teaching me my first lesson: Our patients are humans too.

In medicine, we like to think that our patients are invincible, that with enough medication, we can defeat mortality. And yet, medicine is at its best when it recognizes our shared mortality, our collective humanity. It is then, in that moment of humility, that we can begin the process of compassionately caring, the process of healing the wounds that reside below the surface. To achieve this, our patients need real heroes. These heroes are not found flying through the sky or on the movie screens wearing vintage boots and red capes. They take the shape of ordinary people—like the doctor who checks in on his patient one last time before signing out for the night, to promise that everything is going to be okay in the morning. They take the shape of the resident who holds his patient's hand until he falls asleep. And, for Andriy, they take the shape of the aunt willing to travel around the world in order to save the life of a young boy.

It was a cold, gray morning in Boston, as I stepped off the subway line and made my way through the unusually busy Saturday morning commotion outside the train station. Balancing on the tips of my freshly-shined brown shoes, I felt out of place as I peered over the heads around me, into the sea of red and blue hats, scarves, and wool sweaters emblazed with the letters of the alumni's alma maters. It was only three hours away from kickoff of the 131st Harvard-Yale Game. The air was buzzing. One could feel the electricity and excitement that permeated the crowd. Wherever I turned, I was greeted with smiles, cheers, chants, and quick "hellos," as former classmates rushed to catch the next train to Alewife. I found myself pushing against the herd, struggling to make my way through the masses to the towering glass building that loomed overhead. The lobby was empty and dark. Only the soft, gray light that had managed to sneak through the clouds filled the room. A new Christmas tree and wagon overflowing with presents had been placed behind the security desk to welcome the holiday season. Behind the large desk, the security guard smiled and greeted me. We spoke only briefly during my last visit, but I remember being struck by his charming personality. He was young, no more than 25 years old. Dressed in a freshly-starched security uniform, and equipped with a shining smile, he was just what the hospital needed on that cold, gray morning. As we spoke, I unzipped my bag, pulled out my carefully-folded white coat, pinned my security badge to my lapel, and gathered my thoughts, as I prepared for my second visit with Andriy. I said goodbye to the security guard and walked to the elevators around the corner.

The doors opened onto the seventh floor. I was the only person in sight. I looked around for the entrance to the ward. Anyone watching would have known that I was a first-year medical student. Fortunately, I was alone and my ignorance went unnoticed. The entrance to Andriy's floor was behind a large play area, filled with toys, a pool table, games, a giant television, outfitted with a lifetime supply of video games, and a snug couch calling for someone to sit down and play. It seemed the perfect oasis for a child, a safe-haven from the struggles that lived behind the doors in front of me. I wondered how many children had sat on that couch, how many parents had stood where I stood, looking on as their child played. How many lives had been saved by heroes like Dr. Grove? Probably too many to count.

Dr. Grove is one of those special people who have the ability to heal the soul merely by his presence. His smile and calm tone of voice exude a sense of peace that I struggle to adequately describe with words. He had only interacted with me on three other occasions, yet, when I ran into him in the ward that morning, he instantly put me at ease and welcomed me back to the hospital with a bright smile. He introduced me to his colleague Greg, a vascular surgeon whose graying hair spoke of the years of stress and training he had endured. Greg was preparing to leave Boston and move with his family to a new job in Pittsburgh. Expensive Boston real-estate prices and an exciting offer had convinced him to make the move and start a new chapter in his life. For a brief second, I wondered what my life would look like in 10 years, at the end of residency. I unconsciously ran my fingers through my hair as I thought about the white hairs that would surely come with time.

Outside Andriy's room, behind a long desk, was a group of nursing students whispering and laughing with one another. They looked happy and excited to take care of Andriy and the other patients on the floor. Andriy was lying in bed, watching a movie, while Aleksandra zipped around the room organizing his clothes. After checking in and saying hello, Dr. Grove left me with Aleksandra, so I could start my second visit. My goal, as he recommended, was to learn more about the social issues surrounding Andriy's case. "Where do I begin?" I thought.

The past night, he had woken up at 4 a.m., which explained why they both looked so exhausted. He was recovering from a Monday operation on his head, and his trach was still where it had been when I last visited. Pain from the surgeries and the tubes dangling from his elbows made it hard to sleep. Aleksandra shared that narcotics were necessary to fight off his most severe pain. With those drugs came more sleepiness and fatigue, so they tried to avoid them whenever possible. On a good note, his diet and appetite were improving. Aleksandra was sneaking in gourmet Russian food from a nearby store. I can only imagine how good it must have tasted after weeks of bland hospital meals. With food, of course, comes strength, and Andriy was improving with his physical therapy exercises. He could walk, but doing so independently was still a struggle.

I asked about future surgeries, but was unsurprised to learn that Aleksandra was unsure how much longer they would need to stay, how many more operations awaited them, or even what medications he was taking. Understandably, the language barrier must have been a major obstacle for the care team. I had met the translator on one of my first visits, but could only imagine how much was lost in translation, even when the translator was around. Even I was struggling to communicate my straightforward questions in an understandable way that a non-English speaker could understand. The sheer stress of being in a foreign place, alone, must have been overwhelming. Andriy had also made little progress in his English. He could only communicate pain, hunger, or bathroom needs in English. Yet, there he was, smiling and giggling as "Daddy Day Care" played on the television overhead.

I remembered watching "Daddy Day Care" when I was just beginning high school, back home in New Jersey. It is a comedy in which Eddie Murphy plays the role of a recently unemployed father who starts a day care service with friends to make money. The story hits on the importance of family, prioritizing children, and caring for others. While still unclear, I was beginning to suspect that Andriy's childhood differed starkly from that of the children on the television screen. Aleksandra reiterated that she had had no choice but to come to the United States, not only because she loved Andriy and felt a responsibility toward him, but also because Andriy's mother would not come. Communication with his mother seemed infrequent, and Aleksandra stated that they had not spoken to her sister that week. I wanted to probe further, but decided to save my questions for another time. Instead, I asked about friends in America. She admitted that Andriy was mostly alone. Another patient from Ukraine had arrived, but another child with whom he had become friends left at the same time. People were passing in and out of his life. The happy image of Eddie Murphy holding his son's hand was an ideal that Andriy may never have experienced. He did not need to understand English to appreciate what it means for a child to have parents who love him and are there for him. Only Aleksandra was a constant in his life.

Aleksandra, in many respects, was the victim of two simultaneous battles. The first was one she was fighting with her own hands, in Andriy's hospital room every day. The second was one she could not fight, but could only watch on the television screen as events unfolded. When Russia's parliament approved President Putin's request to use force to protect Russian interests, this was followed with a referendum to absorb Crimea. In response, Ukraine's acting President ordered the military to begin operations against pro-Russian terrorists in the East. Among those Ukrainian men called to serve was Aleksandra's husband. Meanwhile, she was left behind with a child who Ukrainian doctors said had zero chance for survival— unless he went to America. The conflict, which was separating nations, had now also separated her from her husband, who had to fight for his country instead of coming to Boston to fight alongside her in Andriy's battle. She admitted to praying for her husband's safety. Her facial expressions and words conveyed her stress and worry. Though she communicated with him, she missed him, longed to return home, and prayed that he would be waiting for her when she arrived. But Aleksandra had no time to nurse her own wounds. She was busy tending to her nephew's. Maybe this was a good thing for her. Maybe it helped her cope. She could not help her husband, but at least she could help someone she loved.

Across from his bed was a makeshift calendar with pictures of different activities taped next to each day of the week. Aleksandra kept a strict schedule of psychiatrist, nutritionist, physical therapy, and doctors' meetings. She admitted to me that many of the services taped on that calendar might not be available back in Ukraine. They lived 15 minutes away from a hospital that could not cater to the broad spectrum of needs Andriy required. It was also unclear how they would pay for any services or his return trips to the United States for continued treatment at the hospital. Yet, this insecurity only propelled her forward. She had made a habit of sleeping in Andriy's room at night in an arm chair, rather than going to her hotel room. Andriy would call her at 3 or 4 a.m. when she was away, so she cut her losses and reasoned it would be best for both of them if she slept by his side. That way neither of them would wake up alone in the middle of the night.

While Aleksandra's hardships as a caretaker may easily go overlooked by the healthcare system, they are not unusual. Patients like Andriy require longterm care, broadly defined as care needed to survive when mental and physical disabilities inhibit daily activities. These activities include dressing, bathing, eating, and using the bathroom. Despite the existence of nursing homes, assisted living, adult foster and day care, home healthcare agencies, and other sources of formal care, most care is provided informally by family and friends. The burden for caretakers takes on physical, emotional, and financial proportions. There are over 44 million unpaid caretakers in America. They are over-represented by low-income individuals and most are women. The psychological and social impact is equally great. Among Alzheimer's caregivers, 80 percent report high levels of stress, and at least half report depression. The toll includes a greater incidence of illness, decreased life expectancy, and reduced quality of life.

These thoughts filled my mind as I gathered my belongings and prepared to leave. I thanked Aleksandra for her time. She turned to me, smiled, and unexpectedly said, "Thank you for your time, for coming and listening to us." I was only a first-year medical student, but her smile and the look in her eyes suggested that I was making a difference, however small it may be. As I turned for the door, I looked out the window to see the sky still gray, with that ominous look of winter coming. I commented on the inevitable snow that awaited us, and Aleksandra's face lit up. "Andriy can't wait to see the snow!" she exclaimed, as she looked affectionately at him and pointed at the sky, while she translated in Russian. They would be spending their first Christmas in America. Despite all they had been through, they managed to turn what normally makes Bostonians gloomy into something they could look forward to. Every cloud has its silver lining, I thought. Our patients are amazing at reminding us of that.

It was a good thing I brought an umbrella. The rain was starting to come down. As I walked through the entrance to the hospital, I looked down at my watch, which read 10 a.m. Right on time, I thought to myself. I shook the rain off my jacket and umbrella. I dried my shoes on the mat and walked up to the front desk, where I exchanged a few friendly words with the security guard. The familiarity of the place made me feel more at home and confident, as I prepared to go upstairs. It was as I had expected. Quiet and empty. The seventh-floor play area was filled with the idle toys that had greeted me the previous

Saturday. Recalling my weekday visit to the hospital in October, I felt relieved that Aleksandra had been comfortable with me visiting on the more peaceful weekends. Saturdays were Andriy's good days. I recalled the calendar hanging on his bathroom door, each day filled with school lessons, psychologist meetings, physical therapy (PT), a lunch break, more PT, play time with other children, and then more school, before a break for the rest of the day. I made a mental note to stop by again during the week before he left for Ukraine.

When I entered the ward, I found some nurses seated outside Andriy's room, which was still draped with curtains. I could barely make out the glimpse of a shadow between the cracks. Aleksandra was awake and getting the room organized. The nurses recommended I wait outside. A sigh of relief escaped as I stretched my arms and legs. It had been a long week of classes. After a few minutes passed, I pulled out my computer and searched for news on the Ukrainian conflict. Why bother, I thought, as I scrolled through the pages. The conflict seemed so distant and intangible, as I sat comfortably in my white coat, thousands of miles away from the violence. Yet, war always manages to find its way into even the most sacred places, when you least expect it. It is ruthless, unbiased, and makes no distinctions between its victims. When I saw Aleksandra approaching from the corner of my eye, the conflict, for a brief second, suddenly felt very real.

"Are you coming?" she asked. "Of course!" I replied. I had been looking forward to seeing how Andriy had improved. She told me to wait where I was while she used the bathroom. He was getting ready and needed another 15 minutes. Waiting for Aleksandra, I reflected on the journey they had endured. When Andriy arrived in July he was barely alive. His doctors at home had given him a slim chance of survival. But, somehow, our "Superman" overcame the odds. Not only that, but he did so in a foreign country, far from friends, family, and the little things in life that make us feel at home.

While in mid-thought, Aleksandra returned and beckoned, "Follow me." Andriy was just waking up, the bags under his eyes still visible from a long night's rest. Aleksandra exclaimed, "I told him, Eugene is coming today! You can't sleep in, you need to wake up!" Andriy smiled and waved at me from beneath his blanket, while Aleksandra laughed. I was touched to think that they had been looking forward to my visit. I thought back to last weekend when Aleksandra thanked me for caring about them and taking the time to follow their story.

A movie was playing overhead. It was "Rush Hour," and Jackie Chan was darting across the screen, drawing intermittent giggles from Andriy, as he lay snug underneath his teddy bear blanket. I could tell that he was improving every day. He could now walk around the hospital independently and roll around in his bed, though this would quickly tangle him up in his cables, and bring out scorning words from his aunt. He also looked much better since the last visit: His smile was brighter and his face looked fuller. Aleksandra's Russian food was having its effect. She also mentioned that he was eating lots of apples and other fruit. I could tell how proud and grateful she was that he was doing this well. In between her words, she stretched her arm out and ran her fingers through the tufts of hair that were growing back on his head. The skin under his hair was healing and his scalp looked healthier. While she massaged the hairs between her finger tips, she nodded toward his picture on the bathroom door. He was a handsome boy.

His fingers were also getting better, and he had regained some dexterity. When Aleksandra brought a straw and a bottle of milk over, he gulped it down. His tracheostomy was gone but his face contorted with pain after each gulp. I wondered if this was due to his surgeries or the aftermath of his burns. It was obvious that this recovery would not have been possible without Aleksandra's incredible sacrifice and dedication. She took his splints off at night, lubricated his skin with special creams, exercised with him when the therapists could not make it, monitored his diet, put on his clothes, changed his diapers, and repositioned the many monitors dangling from his body, so he could move around and sleep. Meanwhile, she juggled the anxiety of what awaited them back home.

When I asked her to expand on her concerns, she said that, in her opinion, the people at home would not understand his condition, and she expressed fear that he might not make it in such an environment. She forbade him to talk with any friends from home while hospitalized. His call with his parents last week was an exception. She was uncertain how children would respond at school. He had completed three years of schooling before the accident. Her hope was to return in February, allow him to readjust to life there, and ultimately enroll him back in school by September. His mother had also promised to return from Italy by then to help.

I was confused by Andriy's relationship with his mother and the obvious tension between her and Aleksandra. Why did she not come to America? After all, it was her child, not Aleksandra's. Why was she in Italy and not back in Ukraine preparing for his return? Why did Aleksandra have to suffer so much? As if reading my thoughts, she said she had no choice. Moreover, she said, "I cannot have children; I have to take care of him now." Then she added, as if predicting the future, "I hope his mother does not have more children." I wanted to probe further, but was fearful of causing any more anxiety.

She also made it clear on multiple occasions that she was desperate for them to leave the hospital. She missed her husband and was overwhelmed by the calls from home for updates, which only left her feeling sadder. With the exception of some Ukrainian friends who stopped by, she was otherwise alone. Yet, as she leaned over Andriy, smiling and fixing his clothes, one would never guess. Like some of the doctors I had met at the hospital, she had that special ability to heal the soul merely by her presence. She hid her anxieties so well behind her smile, radiant blue eyes, and shining blond hair. She and Andriy seemed so happy together. One would never guess that she was his aunt.

While I stood beside his bed, talking to Aleksandra as she did her work on Andriy, I realized that, despite her broken English, we had spoken without saying anything at all, understood one another without a translator in the room, and forged a friendship that brought value to both of our lives.

On my next visit, just before Christmas, I arrived to find a familiar scene: Aleksandra lovingly attending to her nephew, while he lay quietly in bed watching the television. After our usual smiles and hellos, Aleksandra continued her work. She replaced his shirt, checked on his bandages, and showed me the outcome of his latest surgery. On his back was a new white patch, centered over his spine and stretching across the middle of his back. Despite some groans and whining, as Aleksandra applied some cold lubricant to his skin, he otherwise was in good spirits and looked well.

I asked Aleksandra, "What does he want to become when he grows up?" "A doctor,"she answered with a big smile. I was ecstatic and told her that he would become a fine physician. We discussed the possibilities, despite his handicaps, and I noted that some of the healthcare workers at the hospital were also burn survivors. She smiled and looked fondly toward Andriy. Sensing an opportunity, I asked her about her plans when she goes home. "I want to become a nurse," she said. She added that this would help her take care of her nephew and would make both of their lives easier. I told her that, after 6 months of caring for him, she had already earned her nursing license. I tried to imagine their future. Their story was incredible and it was heartening to know that he would always have her by his side during his journey. Her dedication was unparalleled and unexpected for an aunt. I was confused why she felt so obliged to sacrifice the opportunity to have children of her own to take care of her sister's child. As if knowing that it would be my last chance to inquire, I reopened the conversation about his accident and asked, "Where was the barn that caught on fire?" "It was my barn," she answered.

I promised to come back after Christmas break. As Aleksandra translated each sentence, Andriy turned his gaze toward me, nodded his head for a quick second, and then returned his attention to the television screen. As I started to stand, I noticed the "Spiderman" blowup in the corner of the room. I promised to bring him another souvenir to add to his growing Spiderman collection.

When I returned from winter break, Dr. Grove was already one month into his deployment in Afghanistan. Andriy had gotten his wish and was moved out of the hospital. Despite Dr. Grove's best efforts to assist me and connect me with Dr. Piedmont, to facilitate another visit, I never saw Andriy again. If I knew that I would never again see this brave boy waving and smiling back at me from his wheelchair as I left the room that last day, I would have thanked them again for the hundredth time, wished them well with their future, and offered to keep in touch. As I replay that day in my head, my patient is back home with his aunt, and hopefully his mother, adjusting to his new reality.

My journey with Andriy gave me a greater appreciation for things that cannot be fully understood by reading the pages of a textbook. My experience was particularly meaningful since Andriy reminded me of myself, thirteen years ago, when I too was a patient sitting in a hospital room, recovering from a cardiac ablation surgery to treat my supraventricular tachycardia (SVT). The successful operation forever changed my life after years of physical struggle.

I like to think that things happen for a reason, and that my placement with Andriy was deliberate. Maybe it was meant to remind me of where my own life journey began. Ultimately, I hope that my 8-year-old patient benefited from this experience as much as I did. If I ever have the privilege of crossing paths with him again, I will share with him an important lesson that I learned from my medical experience: There are two ways of living—one as if nothing in life is a miracle and one as if everything is.

> The mediocre teacher tells. The good teacher explains. The superior teacher demonstrates. The great teacher inspires.
>
> — William Arthur Ward

Epilogue: Beginnings

LISA MAYER, EDM, NANCY ORIOL, MD, ROBERT C. STANTON, MD, KATHARINE TREADWAY, MD

Everything matters. This is true of many situations in life, but particularly so in patient care. Factors such as the nutrition the patient receives, the extent to which their healthcare team operates as a team, and the physical environment of a hospital room, not to mention their own life situation: financial stability, social support, cultural background; *all* of it is important. If *everything* matters, how should we approach the education of a medical student in the first year? How can we hope to improve the lament of patients exposed to a healthcare system that so often seems dispassionate and uncaring? How can we teach our students to be aware of the entirety of a patient's case, including the life-baggage with which the patient walks into the examination room? How can we encourage thoughtful introspection? How can we prepare them for the ceaseless stream of new information they will need to assimilate during their career in medicine?

These were some of the questions the Harvard Medical School faculty was grappling with in 2003, during a review of its curriculum. The retired HMS dean, Dr. Daniel Tosteson, held strong opinions on the subject of medical education:

> *"Medicine begins in philosophy and philosophy ends in medicine." I would urge them to develop a personal philosophy that would sustain a professional lifetime of learning medicine. I would tell them that if they succeeded in formulating and practicing such a philosophy, the goal of the educational program would be met, and that if they failed in the effort, we would have failed, no*

matter how much knowledge they accumulated while at Harvard Medical School.

Amidst the discussion of curricular reform, he suggested that the student could follow a patient during their first year and "write a book." And so the "Mentored Clinical Casebook Project" was designed, as an experiment at first, to see if we could give our students a useful foundation for what would follow, both in medical school and in their future medical practice.

At a time in their life when the student is more like a patient than a physician, we wanted them to experience a patient's encounters with health care, by accompanying them to medical appointments, visiting them if hospitalized, and seeing them at home (at least once during the year). They observe what it is like for a patient whose first language is not English to navigate the labyrinth of a large urban hospital, and to try to decipher the "medical speak" of their specialist physicians, or what it feels like for a lonely, single person to undergo an HIV AIDs test in an inner-city clinic and wait anxiously for the results. They observe surgery, chemotherapy, birth, or conversations on end-of-life questions.

In designing the course, our hope was that this immersion into the life of one patient, at an impressionable point in their education, would inoculate them against the pushback of a system that sometimes favors capacity over care. And the backdrop for these real-life encounters is the science the student is taught during their first year. Their respective patient brings to life what they learn in lecture and tutorial, infused with the context of that person's whole existence. The casebook also serves as a journal, where students can record personal reflections about entering the medical profession; and it provides a rationale for significant mentorship from faculty—often experts a first-year student would not typically have the opportunity to meet.

More than half of our faculty mentors sign up repeatedly, because it is rewarding to help a student at the start of his or her medical career, and because it can include a tangible benefit for their patient. Some find that their patients with chronic illness are in better health when they are working with our students. At the beginning of the year, the students are perplexed as to why anyone would allow them such a personal look into their lives during a time of illness. Patients report that they get great pleasure out of feeling they are helping "their medical student" become a better physician. And those with a terminal illness find it comforting that their situation may help a young person become a better doctor.

The patient serves as a bridge between the science studied in the classroom and the work observed in a clinical setting. The study of the disease, and the basic science behind it, is the starting point for the student's inquiry, introduced by the faculty mentor, who points the student in the direction of relevant articles and recent research. Meanwhile, the student begins to get to know the patient and the circumstances of his/her life. By learning all they can about one patient, the student encounters the need to integrate the relevant information drawn from various bodies of knowledge, e.g., the physical, biological, and social sciences and the humanities. The unusual opportunity to visit the patient at home, meet family members, accompany them to clinical appointments, or spend time with them in the hospital allows the student exposure to the broad range of factors that affect a patient's care. Through the examination of a single patient, and the study of all the aspects of the person's illness, the student is able to explore how it all fits together: from the molecular basis of the disease to the treatment, the psychological impact, the relationship of the patient's support systems, and financial implications—and everything else that can hinder or facilitate a desired outcome. It is this essential illustration of the big picture that allows them a structure from which to consider and address specific issues in their patients.

Students are assigned randomly to a clinical mentor. The reason for this is that one of the key lessons of the project is that it does not matter what the primary issue presented by the patient may be, that for each person, the myriad aspects of the life of that individual will affect their illness, treatment, and success. No matter what the predominant condition involved, that student will become aware of many other factors materially pertaining to their patient.

Each faculty member handles the matching of student and patient differently. Some choose to meet the student alone first and then determine a suitable patient. Others meet the student for the first time on the day they will introduce them to their patient. And for others, the student is given several files and asked to choose the person with whom they would be most interested in working. Once the student meets the patient, the two of them determine the frequency and occasion of their subsequent meetings. Some patients prefer to meet the student in something other than a clinical setting, e.g., one of our patients routinely met his student in his office.

However, most are comfortable having the student accompany them to clinical appointments, to the extent their class schedule allows; and students learn considerably from these encounters. They sit with their patient in waiting rooms, observe as they absorb medical terminology and difficult diagnoses, and keep them company during long, boring, chemotherapy sessions. If patients are hospitalized, they visit them there, representing a different kind of visitor: one less than a physician, more than a friend; someone keenly interested in the patient's case, but more informed than the average acquaintance or family member, and extremely interested in their success, but not directing their care. Students also visit the patient at home at least once during the year. These are extremely instructive interactions, and the students often meet family members so they can integrate a fuller picture of the patient's social support. Sometimes the home visits become a fairly frequent event. One elderly patient, who felt uneasy in clinical settings, would routinely have the student for dinner to discuss his life and his health.

Mentors are guided into choosing patients with somewhat chronic issues, as we want the student to have more than one clinical interaction during the year. Several of our mentors are surgeons, and their students (remember, they are in their first year of medical school) are treated to dramatic 10-hour days in the OR, sometimes concluding with the physician's evening visit to the family to give the post-operative report.

Surgery isn't required to provide drama, however. And students have been motivated to go to all sorts of lengths to be helpful in their patient's care. One student, mystified by the fact that his teenaged patient's diabetes was much better controlled while home in the summer with his extended family than during the school year, when he lived in Boston, spent spring break traveling to the Caribbean to visit the patient's grandparents and observe his life there. The student developed a very helpful theory for the patient's doctor here in Boston.

Without the necessity of long-distance travel, there are hundreds of examples of ways in which students positively help their patients. At the start of the year, they are baffled by the question of why anyone would let them into their life at what is, by definition, a difficult time. They don't yet understand that, by simply being there for the patient, they are providing a service most of us crave. Through the act of following the patient, listening, and paying attention to them, the students are giving a great and sometimes healing gift, which many come to realize by the end of the school year. One of our repeat mentors routinely assigns the same patient to our students as his Casebook patient. This is because he finds this patient does much better controlling his chronic condition during the months he is involved with the course. The reason is similar to what is behind the success of chronic disease management programs initiated by insurance companies. Kaiser Permanente published a study in 2010, outlining the benefits to heart disease patients of periodic intervention by personal nurses and clinical pharmacy specialists. The same value is derived by patients with diabetes, cancer, or other chronic diseases that require adherence to a schedule of medication, diet plan, or exercise.

Patients who volunteer to allow a first-year student shadow their medical life are often motivated by a desire to educate and help the student become a better doctor. Some, with terminal illness, wish to feel their experience facing end-of-life will result in something positive. Patients sometimes refer proudly to "my Harvard medical student" when introducing the student to their friends or family. And, for patients who subsequently pass away, students often hear from family members that the period during which they were involved with the course was enormously meaningful to the ailing patient.

As an elective course, the enrolled students are self-selected. They know, at the outset, that they will be expected to write a scholarly report of their experience, so the course tends to attract students who are not afraid to write. But that does not preclude our offering support for their writing effort throughout the year. In addition to their clinical mentor, students are also assigned to another faculty member in the role of Project Advisor. Groups of four students meet with their Project Advisor during the year, and these sessions serve as a writing course. It is in these meetings that the students share their experiences in the Casebook Project and, as they begin drafting the casebook, they share excerpts and critique each other. Their Project Advisor not only guides the writing but points the student in the direction of other resources they might follow, as they look into the diseases or conditions of their case. It is another example of a mentoring opportunity not usually afforded to a first-year student, and these relationships often last beyond the student's first year.

We aim for half of the clinical mentors each year to be renewals, in order always to have a group of seasoned mentors, augmented by newly enthusiastic teachers. Despite the fact that this entire endeavor is voluntary, the faculty is always eager to participate again.

These busy, practicing clinicians eagerly sign up year after year. They report that, in addition to learning more about their patient, and therefore able to be more helpful, the experience reminds them what it was like when they were in their first year of medical school. The enthusiasm for medicine that first-year students exude is wonderful and contagious.

In Year 1, students are hit with a tremendous amount of information to learn in class and in the lab, and all the while they are grappling with their self-image, and how it can be reconciled with the physician they will ultimately become. In addition, they are drawn to training that will ultimately lead to their being able to help people; yet, in the first year, their contact with patients is usually limited. The Casebook Project gives them a place to express both concern and questions about the larger, existential issues that worry an undergraduate medical student. It gives them a construct in which to develop mentoring relationships with faculty they would almost never ordinarily encounter in their first year, and it gives them entrée into a patient's life that they will most certainly never have again. This all happens at a time when they are receptive, hungry to take in the totality of health care. In the early years of running the course, one of the students expressed surprise that the course was an elective, as opposed to a requirement, saying "I thought this *was* what medical school was supposed to be!"

One student put it this way, at the end of his first year:

Relationships between doctor and patient frequently develop while neither one is actively processing the details of an agenda, but rather becoming engrossed in dialogue. Moments that are appropriate for the activity of reflection punctuate a longitudinal interaction, especially towards the conclusion of an interaction that has spanned many themes. Reflection becomes the sine qua non *for organizing and interpreting a diverse array of information, such as that garnered through the Mentored Clinical Casebook Project. . . . I, frankly, I cannot imagine going through the first year of medical school without participating in such a project.*

311

During the year, there are also three all-class meetings. In the fall, we explore the topic of how to relate to the patient; in the spring, there is a session on writing about medicine; and in late spring, an evening session during which the students give brief, oral presentations on their experience. This gives the class a broader view of the illnesses and conditions being explored.

Another student explained his experience this way:

> *The difficulty of this project has been learning how to think about another human being, to understand the complex connections within a person, and his or her complex connections to the world at large. I think this is a factor of time spent listening and time spent reflecting. In struggling with this, somehow things fell into place, and I hope I was able to gain insight into (my patient's) life. I have realized that the struggle itself is the source of understanding.*

All in all, it is a lot to ask of a first-year medical student. But because the opportunity comes at exactly the right time, we have found our students gain at least as much as they give. They find it fascinating that the river of the presenting illness leads them down all sorts of tributaries.

The overarching goal of the Mentored Clinical Casebook Project is to create an environment that encourages students to learn how to learn; to assume personal responsibility for learning what they need to know when they need to know it; to encourage a love for learning. These essays demonstrate the achievement of this goal.

About the Editors

Susan E. Pories, MD, FACS is an Associate Professor of Surgery at Harvard Medical School and the Medical Director of The Hoffman Breast Center at Mount Auburn Hospital in Cambridge, Massachusetts. Dr. Pories is the Associate Co-Director of the Arts and Humanities Initiative at HMS. She was awarded the 2010 A. Clifford Barger Excellence in Mentoring Award by Harvard Medical School.

Samyukta Mullangi, MD, MBA is a third-year resident at the University of Michigan. She graduated with a dual MD-MBA degree from Harvard Medical School and Harvard Business School, and is interested in healthcare technology and delivery system innovation.

Aakash Kaushik Shah, MD is an emergency room doctor at Rutgers-Robert Wood Johnson University Hospital in New Jersey. He also serves as a health policy advisor to several state legislators and non-profits. His policy work focuses on responses to the opioid crisis, outreach and enrollment for health insurance, and access to healthcare. He obtained his MD from Harvard Medical School, MBA and MSc from Oxford University as a Rhodes Scholar, and BA and BS from Ursinus College.

Mounica Vallurupalli, MD is a fellow in hematology and oncology at Dana-Farber Cancer Institute and Massachussetts General Hospital. She completed her medical degree at Harvard Medical School, graduating magna cum laude. She went on to train in internal medicine at Brigham and Women's Hospital. She plans to pursue a career in academic oncology and hopes to continues to use the lessons in narrative medicine that she learned as a first-year medical student to better understand the illness narratives of her patients.

Course Faculty

Lisa Mayer, EdM is the Executive Director of the Giovanni Armenise-Harvard Foundation, which supports basic science research. In addition, she has been involved in the Mentored Clinical Casebook Project since 2002, when the late Dean Emeritus Daniel Tosteson convened the Steering Committee to develop this course for first-year Harvard medical students. It has been extraordinarily rewarding for her to work with students at this early stage in their education, and to see the exceptional insights the students glean during their experience with patients and mentors.

Nancy Oriol, MD is Associate Professor of Anesthesia at Beth Israel Deaconess Medical Center, Lecturer on Global Health and Social Medicine and Faculty Associate Dean for Community Engagement in Medical Education at Harvard Medical School.

Robert C. Stanton, MD is the Chief of the Kidney and Hypertension Section at the Joslin Diabetes Center, a staff physician at the Beth Israel Deaconess Medical Center, and an Associate Professor of Medicine at Harvard Medical School. Dr. Stanton is a teacher, clinician, and does both basic and clinical research. He has received three Honorary Professorships and he received a major lifetime-achievement teaching award for sustained excellence in teaching from Harvard Medical School.

Katharine Treadway, MD is the Gerald S. Foster Academy Associate Professor of Medicine at Harvard Medical School. She is a primary care doctor at Massachusetts General Hospital and teaches several courses at the medical school

Student Authors

Adaugo Amobi, MD, MPH is currently completing her residency in Internal Medicine at Massachusetts General Hospital. She received a bachelor's degree in anthropology from Princeton University and completed a dual MD/MPH program at Harvard

Medical School and the Harvard School of Public Health. Ada is passionate about women's health, social justice and violence prevention. She hopes to have a career providing patient-centered clinical care and developing community-based public health interventions.

Kia Byrd is a native of Jackson, Mississippi. She completed her Bachelor of Science degree at Howard University and is now a 4th year MD/MPH candidate with a concentration in health policy at Harvard Medical School and the Harvard T.H. Chan School of Public Health. She hopes to integrate her training in health policy and medicine into a career as both a clinician and advocate, working to expand medical, legal, and social services for vulnerable, disenfranchised women, particularly in the southern United States.

Galina Gheihman, HBSc is an MD Candidate (Class of 2019) in the Pathways Program at Harvard Medical School. Raised in Toronto, she attended the University of Toronto, where she majored in Neuroscience and Psychology. At HMS, Galina is a member of the Student Leadership Committee at the Centre for Primary Care, serving as the editor of the Primary Care Considered Blog and leader of the Communications & Narrative Medicine Subcommittee (C&NM). She is also assistant editor for Fiction and Creative Non-Fiction at thirdspace, an online literary journal.

Carla Heyler grew up in Southern California and later migrated to Atlanta, Georgia, where she graduated from Emory University with a degree in Biology and a formal plan to study medicine. Like many things planned, her path took an unexpectedly different route. The short version is that after completing three years at Harvard, Carla stepped away from medical school with a Masters in Medical Science. The long version is very long, but suffice it to say that the MD part isn't over yet!

Manjinder Singh Kandola is finishing his fourth year at HMS and currently pursuing a MBA at Stanford. He is planning to apply for a residency in internal medicine. Manjinder followed up recently on the patient described in his essay and was thrilled to learn that he ultimately began treatment as recommended, responded very well and is currently in remission.

Janine Knudsen, MD was inspired by her experience getting to know and support a patient through the Mentored Clinical Casebook Project and chose to pursue a career in primary care. After majoring in Public Health Studies at Johns Hopkins University she graduated from Harvard Medical School and completed her training in the Primary Care Track of the NYU Internal Medicine Residency Program. She currently practices as a primary care physician at Bellevue Medical Center in New York City with a focus on improving care for the underserved.

Grace Lee, MD is a general surgery resident at the Massachusetts General Hospital in Boston, MA. She grew up in Maryland, attended college at the Massachusetts Institute of Technology, and received her medical degree from Harvard Medical School. She is interested in colorectal surgery and clinical outcomes research.

Clare Malone grew up in the Chicago suburbs, and then attended Williams College, where she double-majored in biology and French language and literature. She earned a PhD in genetics and certificate in human biology and translational medicine from Harvard University. She is now a postdoctoral research fellow in the pediatric oncology department at Dana Farber Cancer Institute, where she does research on neuroblastoma.

Aleksandra Olszewski, MD is originally from Poland and grew up in southern Wisconsin. She graduated from Harvard Medical School in 2016 magna cum laude with honors in medical education. Currently a pediatric resident at Seattle Children's Hospital, she is interested in medical education, healthcare disparities and ethics.

Ithan Peltan, MD completed a residency in internal medicine at Massachusetts General Hospital, followed by a fellowship in pulmonary and critical care at the University of Washington.

He is now on the faculty at Intermountain Medical Center and the University of Utah in Salt Lake City, where he provides clinical care and teaches in the intensive care unit and conducts clinical research on sepsis and cardiac arrest. He enjoys spending time hiking, swimming, cooking, and reading with his daughter, Coralie, and wife, Quang-Tuyen.

Morgan Prust, MD graduated from Harvard Medical School in 2015 and is currently a neurology resident at Massachusetts General Hospital and Brigham and Women's Hospital.

Priyanka Saha earned her Bachelor's degree in Biology at the Massachusetts Institute of Technology and is currently a medical student at Harvard Medical School. Priyanka was awarded a 2017-2018 Sarnoff Foundation Fellowship through which she conducted research on congenital heart diseases, such as the one affecting the young girl at the center of her essay. Inspired by her interactions with this resilient young girl and other children living with heart defects, Priyanka hopes to become a pediatric cardiologist and to dedicate her career to improving the lives of children with heart disease through clinical practice and research.

Daniel Seible, MD is a senior radiation oncology resident at UC San Diego. He is presently conducting research on improving quality of cancer care for the Hispanic underserved population, and spends his free time enjoying the ocean and outdoors with his wife and two young children.

Davis "Mac" Stephen, MD is a third-year Internal Medicine resident at Vanderbilt University. He received his undergraduate degree from the University of Arkansas in Biology and Anthropology before attending Harvard Medical School where he received his MD as well as an MMSc in global health delivery.

Eugene Vaios, MD, graduated from Harvard College in 2014 with a degree in Neurobiology, Summa Cum Laude with highest honors in field. He is a class of 2019 MD/MBA candidate at Harvard Medical School and Harvard Business School. Eugene's passion is at the intersection of cancer biology and technology innovation.

Ariel Wagner, MD graduated from Princeton University in 2005 with a BA in the Woodrow Wilson School for International and Public Affairs and certificates in Latin American Studies and in African Studies. She was a Peace Corps volunteer in Mali from 2005-2008, where she led health education projects and ran a pediatric malnutrition program. In 2015, she received her MD degree and a Master's degree in Global Health Delivery from Harvard Medical School. She is currently a chief resident at Contra Costa Family Medicine Residency in Martinez, California. Her interests include global health, social justice, care of underserved communities, obstetrics and reproductive health. After residency, she looks forward to a career in rural global health, with an emphasis on clinical care and teaching.

Acknowledgments

This inspiring project, publishing mentored case books written by first year medical students, is an example of how writing about the experience of studying and practicing medicine can lead to powerful shared reflections that teach all of us valuable lessons. We are very grateful to Dean Nancy Oriol, Dr. Kate Treadway, Dr. Robert Stanton, and Lisa Mayer who oversaw the Mentored Casebook Project and helped connect us with students willing to share their incredible essays. We are so appreciative of the mentors who guided the medical students through their very first experiences of "doctoring." And we extend our heartfelt gratitude to the patients who welcomed the students into the most vulnerable parts of their lives.

We are fortunate that Harvard Medical School has been supportive of efforts to bring the arts and humanities into medical student education. As one of the Associate Co-Directors of the Arts and Humanities Initiative at HMS, it has been one of the great joys of my life to see this change in culture take place. Special thanks for this go to David S. Jones, Lisa M. Wong, and many wonderful physicians who are artists as well as doctors.

We owe a debt of gratitude to my wonderful sister Kathy Pories, Executive Editor at Algonquin Books, who gave many helpful suggestions along the way and provided overall guidance. We are delighted that Sue Meyer, such a talented artist, designed our beautiful cover. And we are most grateful to Richard Altschuler, our copyeditor and publisher for believing in the beauty of this collection and helping us bring these compelling stories to a larger audience.

And we appreciate our families for support and love. Aakash thanks his parents, Kaushik and Rupa, brother Kevan, and wife, Romita, whose sacrifices and unwavering support he could not be more grateful for. Mounica thanks her mother, Vasanti, grandfather, Rama Krishna Rao, grandmother, Tulasi, as well as her uncle Rama Chandra Prasad, aunt Vani, cousin Divya, and her extended family for their all-encompassing love and support, and for believing in the beauty of her dreams. I am especially thankful to Christopher, Louie, Bart, Gabe, Erica, Birdie and Lee, Mary Jane, Carolyn, Walter, Mary Ann, and my mother, Muriel.

CPSIA information can be obtained
at www.ICGtesting.com
Printed in the USA
LVHW020056281218
602004LV00001BB/70